LYME DISEASE

DIET COOKBOOK

FOR BEGINNERS

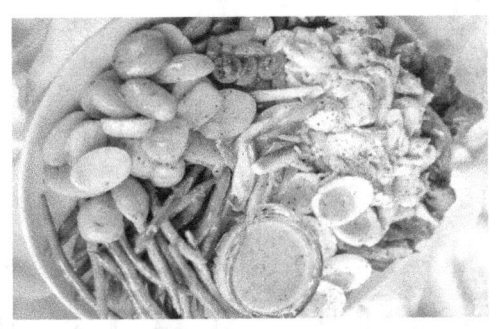

A Beginner's Guide To Lyme Simple Nutritious Recipes And Essential Tips For Managing Tick-Borne Diseases

Thelma Pauley

TABLE OF CONTENT

Introduction

Introduction

Lyme disease, a complicated and sometimes misunderstood illness, presents a lot of difficulties for people who deal with its everyday consequences. Lyme disease may have a far-reaching influence on one's life, causing agonizing exhaustion, chronic pain, and neurological symptoms. In the face of such hardship, developing effective measures for symptom management and enhancing quality of life becomes critical. One such method that has received more attention in recent years is the function of diet in Lyme disease management.

In this introductory chapter, we will investigate the complex link between Lyme disease and food. We look at the scientific knowledge of Lyme disease, its impact on the body, and how nutrition might affect symptom severity and general well-being. We also present the concept of this cookbook, which is a practical guide intended particularly for novices navigating the hurdles of Lyme disease and looking to harness the power of nutrition to help them on their health path.

Lyme disease, caused by the bacterium Borrelia burgdorferi, is usually transmitted to humans by the bite of infected ticks. While the typical indication of Lyme disease is a distinctive bullseye rash, not everyone develops this visual marker. Instead, Lyme disease can present in a variety of ways, from flu-like symptoms in the early stages to more severe and persistent problems if left untreated.

One of the distinguishing qualities of Lyme disease is its tendency to mimic other ailments, resulting in misdiagnosis and delayed treatment for many people. The bacteria that cause Lyme disease can enter multiple internal systems, including the neurological system, joints, heart, and skin, causing a wide range of symptoms. Symptoms may include weariness, joint discomfort, muscular pains, cognitive problems, neurological difficulties, and mood swings, among others.

The insidious character of Lyme disease stems from its capacity to avoid the body's immune response and develop chronic infection, resulting in continuing inflammation and tissue damage. As a result, people with Lyme disease frequently struggle to manage their symptoms and maintain a high quality of life. Traditional treatment methods often include antibiotics to combat the bacterial infection, but many patients feel that this is insufficient to address the entire range of their symptoms.

In recent years, academics and physicians have begun to acknowledge the possible role of nutrition in Lyme disease care. While dietary treatments cannot cure Lyme disease or substitute medical therapy, they can significantly improve general health and well-being. Individuals with Lyme disease can improve their nutritional condition by fueling their bodies with nutrient-dense meals and reducing inflammatory triggers.

Several fundamental concepts govern the creation of a Lyme-friendly diet. The emphasis is on full, unprocessed meals that supply important nutrients and promote immunological function. A healthful Lyme-friendly diet includes fresh fruits and vegetables, lean meats, healthy fats, and complex carbs. These foods provide a wide range of vitamins, minerals, antioxidants, and phytonutrients that are essential for aiding healing and lowering inflammation.

In addition to eating nutrient-dense meals, people with Lyme disease may benefit from recognizing and avoiding certain dietary triggers that might worsen symptoms. Processed meals, refined sugars, gluten, dairy products, and inflammatory oils are all common causes. Individuals may establish a healing environment within their bodies by eating complete foods and limiting their exposure to harmful triggers.

The Purpose of This Cookbook: To Empower Beginners on Their Dietary Journey

Navigating the world of food limitations and lifestyle modifications may be difficult, especially for individuals who have recently been diagnosed with Lyme disease or are only beginning to consider the significance of nutrition in their health journey. Recognizing this need, this cookbook is intended to be a practical resource for novices looking for advice on how to follow a Lyme-friendly diet.

Our objective is to simplify the dietary change process and equip newcomers with the information, tools, and recipes they need to start their nutritional journey confidently. Whether you're a beginner in the kitchen or just searching for ideas to change up your meals, this cookbook has a plethora of tasty and healthy recipes that are simple, flavorful, and designed to help you achieve your health objectives.

Throughout the pages of this cookbook, you'll find a range of breakfast, lunch, supper, snack, and beverage alternatives, all meticulously prepared to adhere to Lyme-friendly nutritional principles. There's something for everyone's taste and preference, from nourishing soups and salads to fulfilling main dishes and decadent desserts. In addition, we offer practical advice for filling your pantry, navigating the grocery store, and modifying recipes to your requirements and tastes.

Remember that you are not alone on this road of self-discovery and growth. By using the power of nutrition and making conscious decisions every day, you can regain control of your health and enhance your well-being in the face of Lyme disease. Allow this cookbook to be your companion and guide as you start on this wonderful and life-affirming journey toward health and vitality.

Chapter 1: Understanding Lyme Disease and Diet

Lyme disease, a multisystemic disorder caused by the spirochete bacteria Borrelia burgdorferi, has become a major public health issue globally. Lyme disease, named after the town of Lyme, Connecticut, where it was discovered in 1975, is largely spread to people by the bite of infected black-legged ticks, sometimes known as deer ticks. Lyme disease is most common in North America, although it has also been documented in Europe, Asia, and other locations.

Complexities of Lyme Disease

Lyme disease is known for its complicated and diverse appearance, making it difficult to identify and treat. The early stage of infection is characterized by flu-like symptoms such as fever, chills, headache, lethargy, and muscular pains, as well as the distinctive erythema migrans rash. However, not all individuals acquire this recognizable rash, resulting in underreporting and misdiagnosis.

If not treated, Lyme disease can develop to the disseminated stage, in which the bacteria spreads throughout the body via the circulation, lymphatic system, and cerebrospinal fluid. This can cause a variety of symptoms including the joints, neurological system, heart, and other organs. Common signs include arthritis, neurological symptoms such as neuropathy and cognitive impairment, heart irregularities, and dermatological problems.

Lyme disease frequently coexists with other tick-borne illnesses, known as coinfections, including Babesia, Anaplasma, Bartonella, and others. Coinfections can aggravate symptoms and complicate therapy, adding to the complexity of Lyme disease care.

Challenges in Diagnosis and Treatment

Lyme disease can be difficult to diagnose owing to its vague symptoms and the few diagnostic tools available. The typical diagnostic strategy is to use serological testing to identify Borrelia burgdorferi antibodies in the blood. However, these tests have limitations, such as sensitivity and specificity fluctuation, which can result in false negatives and positives.

Furthermore, the persistence of symptoms in some patients despite antibiotic therapy has sparked disagreement and contention in the medical community about whether Lyme disease is chronic or persistent. While some experts believe that chronic symptoms are caused by continued infection or immunological dysregulation, others ascribe them to other causes, such as post-treatment Lyme disease syndrome (PTLDS) or other comorbidities.

Lyme disease is normally treated with antibiotics, with the regimen and duration determined by the stage of illness and the presence of coinfections. Early-stage Lyme disease is often treated with oral antibiotics for 2-4 weeks, such as doxycycline, amoxicillin, or cefuroxime. In situations of widespread or late-stage illness, intravenous antibiotics may be required for an extended period.

Diet and Lyme Disease Management

In addition to conventional treatment, many Lyme disease patients seek complementary and alternative techniques to manage their symptoms and improve their general health and well-being. Dietary treatment of Lyme disease is one such strategy that has received more attention.

While dietary treatments cannot cure Lyme disease or replace traditional medical therapy, they can supplement current therapies and aid in the body's healing process. The justification for dietary treatments stems from their ability to decrease inflammation, boost immunological function, and increase general health and vitality.

Understanding the Effects of Diet on Inflammation

Inflammation is a defining characteristic of Lyme disease and plays an important role in its development. The immune system's reaction to Borrelia burgdorferi infection initiates an inflammatory cascade, causing tissue damage and symptom development. Chronic inflammation has been linked to the development of Lyme disease and the duration of symptoms in certain people.

The food we eat can either increase or decrease inflammation in our bodies. Processed foods, refined carbohydrates, trans fats, and high levels of omega-6 fatty acids have all been linked to inflammation and an increased risk of chronic diseases. A diet high in whole, unprocessed foods, such as fruits and vegetables, lean proteins, healthy fats, and complex carbs, has anti-inflammatory properties and promotes overall health.

Importance of Nutrient Density

Nutrient density is the concentration of vitamins, minerals, antioxidants, and other vital elements in a particular diet. Nutrient-dense meals give the body the essential components it needs to perform properly and stay healthy and vibrant. In the context of Lyme disease, selecting nutrient-dense meals can assist promote immune function, enhance tissue healing, and reduce inflammation.

Fruits and vegetables are particularly high in vitamins, minerals, and phytonutrients, which aid immune function and decrease inflammation. Leafy greens, berries, citrus fruits, cruciferous veggies, and vividly colored food are especially antioxidant-rich. Including a variety of fruits and vegetables in your diet provides a diverse range of nutrients and supports general health and well-being.

The Role of Macronutrients

In addition to micronutrients, macronutrients such as carbs, proteins, and fats are needed for maintaining health and vitality. However, not all macronutrients are the same, and their quality can have a substantial influence on health consequences.

Carbohydrates are the body's major source of energy, powering cellular functions and facilitating physical activity. However, not all carbs are created equal, and refined carbohydrates like white bread, sugary snacks, and processed meals can cause inflammation and increase the risk of chronic illness. Complex carbs, such as those found in whole grains, legumes, fruits, and vegetables, give long-term energy and help to maintain stable blood sugar levels.

Proteins are the body's building blocks, responsible for tissue repair, immunological function, and hormone synthesis. High-quality protein sources include lean meats, poultry, fish, eggs, dairy products, legumes, nuts, and seeds, which offer vital amino acids and promote overall health. A diversity of protein sources in the diet offers a well-balanced intake of important nutrients while also promoting muscle development, repair, and maintenance.

Fats are essential for maintaining cell structure and function, producing hormones, absorbing nutrients, and regulating inflammation. While some lipids, such as trans fats and saturated fats, can cause inflammation and increase the risk of chronic illness, others, such as monounsaturated fats, polyunsaturated fats, and omega-3 fatty acids, have anti-inflammatory properties and enhance cardiovascular health.

Dietary Concerns for Lyme Disease Patients

Given the complicated interplay between nutrition, inflammation, and Lyme disease, a few dietary concerns are worth considering for Lyme disease patients:

1. Focus on Whole, Unprocessed Foods

Prioritize complete, unprocessed foods high in vitamins, minerals, antioxidants, and phytonutrients. Fill your plate with a mix of fruits, vegetables, lean meats, healthy fats, and complex carbs to promote general health and well-being.

2. Minimize Inflammatory Triggers

Identify and limit your exposure to possible inflammatory triggers such as processed meals, refined sugars, trans fats, gluten, dairy, and certain vegetable oils. These foods have been demonstrated to cause inflammation and may worsen symptoms in certain Lyme disease patients.

3. Stay Hydrated

Hydration is essential for detoxification, cellular function, and general health. Aim to drink lots of water. To stay hydrated during the day, drink hydrating liquids such as herbal teas, coconut water, and infused water.

4. Support Gut Health

The gut is critical for immune function and inflammatory management, thus Lyme disease patients should prioritize gut health. To promote a healthy microbiome, eat probiotic-rich foods like yogurt, kefir, sauerkraut, and kimchi. Include prebiotic foods like garlic, onions, leeks, and asparagus to support good gut bacteria.

5. Focus on Anti-inflammatory Foods

Include a variety of anti-inflammatory items in your diet to reduce inflammation and promote general health. Omega-3 fatty acids, which may be found in fatty fish, flaxseeds, chia seeds, and walnuts, have powerful anti-inflammatory properties and may help lessen symptoms in Lyme disease patients. Similarly, spices like turmeric, ginger, and cinnamon have anti-inflammatory qualities and may be used in foods and beverages to boost immune function and reduce inflammation.

6. Consider Individual Sensibilities

When creating a Lyme-friendly diet, take into account your body's specific sensitivities and food preferences. Certain meals may be healthy for some people, but they might cause problems in others. Keep a food journal to document your diet and identify any trends or correlations between certain meals and symptoms. Consider working with a healthcare professional or registered dietitian who specializes in Lyme disease to create a personalized nutrition plan based on your unique requirements and objectives.

In conclusion, the link between Lyme disease and nutrition is complicated and multidimensional, with diet having an important role in immune function, inflammation reduction, and general health and well-being. Individuals with Lyme disease can improve their health by choosing nutrient-dense meals, reducing inflammatory triggers, and taking a holistic approach to nutrition.

In the next chapters, we will look at the practical components of establishing a Lyme-friendly diet, such as meal planning, grocery shopping, and recipe modification. We will also present a choice of tasty and healthy meals made exclusively for those living with Lyme disease, including alternatives for breakfast, lunch, supper, snacks, and drinks that follow Lyme-friendly dietary guidelines.

As you begin your culinary adventure, keep in mind that even minor modifications can have substantial consequences. By taking proactive actions to fuel your body with healthy meals and promote your general health and well-being, you may equip yourself to flourish in the face of Lyme disease. Allow this chapter to serve as a starting point for your dietary research, as well as a reminder of the tremendous impact nutrition can have ave in supporting your overall health.

Chapter 2: Building a Lyme-Friendly Pantry

Creating a Lyme-friendly pantry entails stocking up on foods that promote your health while avoiding those that might exacerbate symptoms. Stock your cupboard with full, unprocessed foods such as fruits and vegetables, lean meats, and healthy fats. Choose gluten-free grains such as quinoa and brown rice, as well as alternative flours like almond or coconut.

Include a variety of herbs and spices for taste, with no added salt or artificial ingredients. Avoid processed meals, sugary snacks, and anything with gluten, dairy, or artificial components. With a well-stocked Lyme-friendly pantry, you'll have everything you need to prepare nutritious meals and support your health goals.

Essential Ingredients for a Lyme-Friendly Diet

The key elements for a Lyme-friendly diet are complete, nutrient-dense meals that promote general health and well-being while reducing inflammation and avoiding possible trigger foods. Here are some crucial foods to incorporate into your Lyme-friendly diet:

1. Vegetable

Fill your plate with a variety of colorful veggies, including leafy greens, broccoli, bell peppers, carrots, and squash. These nutrient-dense meals are high in vitamins, minerals, antioxidants, and fiber, which help the immune system and decrease inflammation.

2. Fruits

Eat a variety of fruits, including berries, citrus fruits, apples, pears, and bananas. Fruits include important vitamins, minerals, and antioxidants, as well as natural sweetness, which can fulfill cravings without the need for processed sweets.

3. Lean Protein

Choose lean protein sources such as chicken, fish, eggs, tofu, tempeh, and lentils. Protein is necessary for muscle repair, immunological function, and hormone synthesis, and consuming lean proteins in your diet promotes general health and energy levels.

4. Healthy Fats

Include avocados, nuts, seeds, and olive oil in your diet. These fats contain vital fatty acids, including omega-3s and monounsaturated fats, which have anti-inflammatory characteristics and promote cardiovascular health.

5. Gluten-Free Grains

Choose gluten-free grains such as quinoa, brown rice, millet, and buckwheat, which include complex carbs for long-term energy and fiber for digestion. Gluten-free grains are appropriate for those who are gluten-sensitive or have celiac disease, both of which are frequent among Lyme disease patients.

6. Alternative Flours

To make gluten-free, grain-free dishes, bake and cook with alternative flour such as almond flour, coconut flour, and cassava flour. These flours include less carbs more protein and healthy fats than regular wheat flour, making them appropriate for Lyme-friendly diets.

7. Herbs and Spices

Use a variety of herbs and spices to flavor your food, including turmeric, ginger, garlic, cinnamon, and rosemary. Herbs and spices not only enhance the flavor of foods, but they also contain powerful antioxidants and anti-inflammatory substances that promote immune function and decrease inflammation.

8. Nondairy Milk Alternatives

Instead of cow's milk, use nondairy alternatives such as almond milk, coconut milk, or oat milk. Non-dairy milk alternatives are lactose-free and can serve as a nutritional and tasty substitute in recipes, smoothies, and drinks.

9. Natural Sweeteners

Use natural sweeteners such as honey, maple syrup, or stevia to sweeten dishes without using processed sugars. These natural sweeteners deliver sweetness in moderation while also adding minerals and health benefits.

10. Canned and Jarred Goods

Keep canned beans, tomatoes, and fish on hand, as well as jarred olives, pickles, and salsa, for quick and easy dinner preparation. Look for selections with a few extra ingredients, and choose low-sodium or no-sugar variants wherever feasible.

By stocking your pantry with these basic items, you'll be able to prepare tasty, nutritious meals that promote your health and well-being while addressing Lyme disease symptoms. Experiment with new recipes and tastes to keep your meals interesting and pleasurable, and don't be afraid to see a healthcare practitioner or registered dietitian for specialized nutrition recommendations based on your specific requirements and preferences.

Tips for Grocery Shopping and Meal Planning

Procuring groceries and devising meal plans are crucial aspects of sustaining a diet suitable for those with Lyme disease. Individuals with Lyme disease can optimize their food selection and meal preparation by implementing strategic purchasing habits and strategies to create balanced and nutritious meals that align with their health objectives. Below are some guidelines for grocery shopping and meal planning:

1. Create a list

Before going to the grocery shop, assess the contents of your pantry, fridge, and freezer, and create a list of necessary products. Categorize your list by dietary groups (such as fruits, vegetables, and proteins) to prevent omissions and streamline your shopping excursion.

2. Follow the Outer Boundary

When browsing the grocery store, concentrate on shopping the perimeter, where you'll discover fresh vegetables, lean meats, dairy substitutes, and other nutritious foods. The interior aisles tend to feature more processed and packaged items, which may not correspond with a Lyme-friendly diet.

3. Choose Whole Foods

Choose whole, unprocessed foods whenever available. Opt for fresh fruits and veggies, lean meats, whole grains, and healthy fats instead of packaged and processed meals with additives, preservatives, and refined sugars.

4. Read Labels Carefully

When buying packaged foods, examine ingredient labels carefully to detect possible trigger items such as gluten, dairy, and artificial additives. Look for items with few ingredients and pick alternatives that are free from added sugars, preservatives, and artificial flavors or colors.

5. Shop Seasonally

Take advantage of seasonal produce, which tends to be fresher, more tasty, and more inexpensive. Seasonal fruits and vegetables are particularly rich in nutrients and may bring diversity to your meals throughout the year.

6. Buy in Bulk

Consider purchasing essential products like grains, legumes, nuts, and seeds in bulk to save money and decrease packaging waste. Store bulk materials in sealed containers to ensure freshness and avoid spoiling.

7. Plan Ahead

Set up a time each week to plan your meals and develop a shopping list based on your planned dishes. Consider aspects such as dietary preferences, nutritional needs, and any forthcoming activities or responsibilities when preparing your meals for the week.

8. Batch Cook

Batch cooking includes making big quantities of food ahead of time and portioning it out for future meals. Choose a day of the week to batch cook fundamental ingredients like grains, meats, and veggies, and store them in the fridge or freezer for quick and efficient meal assembly throughout the week.

9. Use Leftovers Creatively

Repurpose leftovers from prior meals to make new recipes and decrease food waste. For example, leftover roasted veggies may be added to salads, soups, or grain bowls, while cooked grains can be changed into stir-fries, salads, or stuffed peppers.

10. Keep it Simple

Focus on simple, healthful meals that need minimum preparation and cooking time. Choose recipes with short ingredient lists and easy directions to ease the meal planning and preparation process.

11. Incorporate Variety

Aim to incorporate a variety of foods in your meals to ensure you're receiving a wide range of nutrients and tastes. Experiment with different fruits, veggies, meats, grains, and spices to make your meals interesting and pleasurable.

12. Consider Dietary Preferences and Restrictions

Take into account any dietary preferences, limits, or food sensitivities while preparing your meals. Customize recipes to meet your specific requirements and preferences, and don't hesitate to make substitutes or alterations as required.

13. Plan for Snacks

Include healthful snacks in your meal plan to keep hunger at bay between meals. Choose snacks that mix protein, fiber, and healthy fats to deliver sustained energy and satiety. Examples include fresh fruit with nut butter, Greek yogurt with berries, or raw veggies with hummus.

14. Shop Mindfully

Practice mindful shopping by concentrating on buying foods that feed your body and support your health objectives. Avoid impulsive purchases and marketing tricks by adhering to your shopping plan and emphasizing nutrient-dense foods.

15. Stay Flexible

Be flexible and adjustable with your meal planning and buying strategy. Life may be unexpected, and it's normal to divert from your plan periodically or make modifications depending on changing circumstances or preferences.

By applying these recommendations for grocery shopping and meal planning, persons with Lyme disease may simplify the process of selecting healthy foods and making balanced meals that promote their health and well-being. With careful planning, conscientious buying, and imaginative food preparation, keeping a Lyme-friendly diet may become a reasonable and pleasurable part of everyday life.

How to Read Food Labels for Hidden Ingredients

Individuals with Lyme disease must read food labels to discover any hidden components that may cause symptoms or increase inflammation. Many processed and packaged foods contain chemicals, preservatives, and other hidden components that may not be obvious from the product name or packaging. Here are some strategies for reading food labels and identifying hidden components.

1. Begin With The Ingredient List

The ingredient list is a detailed list of all the ingredients in the product, arranged in descending order by weight. Scan the ingredient list for any probable allergens, such as gluten, dairy, soy, or artificial additives. Common trigger elements might include:

- Gluten-containing grains (wheat, barley, and rye).

- Dairy products (milk, cheese, and yogurt).

- Soy and its derivatives (soy lecithin, soybean protein)

- Artificial ingredients (preservatives, colors, flavors)

- Refined sugars and sweeteners (high fructose corn syrup, maltodextrin).

- Trans fats, also known as hydrogenated or partially hydrogenated oils, are a type of fat that undergoes a process called hydrogenation.

2. Check for Allergen Warnings

Food labels must include common allergies such as peanuts, tree nuts, eggs, milk, soy, wheat, fish, and shellfish. These allergies must be mentioned on the ingredient list or in a separate allergy statement. If you have known food allergies or sensitivities, pay special attention to allergy warnings to avoid any unwanted responses.

3. Beware of Hidden Sources

Some substances may be disguised with other

names or designated as derivatives, making them less identifiable to consumers. Gluten, for example, can be disguised as hydrolyzed vegetable protein, malt extract, or modified dietary starch, whilst dairy ingredients might be labeled as whey, casein, or lactose. Familiarize yourself with frequent hidden trigger ingredients and learn to identify their alternate names on food labels.

4. Inspect for additives and preservatives

Processed and packaged foods frequently contain chemicals and preservatives to improve flavor, texture, and shelf life. Ingredients to look for include artificial colors (e.g., Red 40, Yellow 5), artificial tastes (e.g., fake vanilla flavor), and preservatives. These substances may cause inflammation and worsen Lyme disease symptoms.

5. Consider the Source

When choosing packaged goods, consider the ingredients' source and quality. Choose items derived from full, natural components and avoid highly processed or refined meals. Choose organic and non-GMO products wherever feasible to reduce your exposure to pesticides and genetically modified organisms.

6. Pay Attention to Serving Sizes.

When reading food labels, be cautious of serving sizes, since they can be misleading and may not reflect true portion amounts. Consider how much you generally take in one sitting and change the nutritional facts to appropriately analyze the product's nutritious content.

7. Exercise Caution With "Healthy" Claims

Be wary of health claims and marketing gimmicks on food packaging, as they can be deceptive or overstated. The terms "all-natural," "low-fat," or "sugar-free" may not always signal a healthy decision. Instead, study the ingredient list and evaluate the nutritional composition of the product to make an educated judgment about its fit for your dietary requirements.

8. Use the Apps and Resources

Make use of smartphone applications and internet sites that give information about food additives, hidden ingredients, and allergy warnings. These tools can help you rapidly detect possible trigger foods and make smart supermarket shopping decisions.

Individuals with Lyme disease who follow these food label reading recommendations can successfully discover hidden components and make educated decisions to promote their health and well-being. With experience and diligence, traversing the grocery store aisle gets simpler, allowing you to confidently choose items that meet your nutritional needs and tastes.

Chapter 3: Breakfast Recipes

Breakfast is frequently regarded as the most essential meal of the day, giving the fuel and nutrients needed to jumpstart our mornings and keep us going until lunch. A nutritious breakfast can be even more beneficial for those with Lyme disease, helping to promote immune function, normalize blood sugar levels, and control symptoms.

Lyme-friendly breakfast dishes, which emphasize nutrient-dense foods and balanced meals, are a tasty and fulfilling way to get the day started correctly. These breakfast alternatives, which range from robust smoothie bowls overflowing with antioxidants to delicious avocado toast filled with healthy fats, are intended to feed the body and promote overall well-being.

Simple and Nutritious Breakfast Options

1. Greek Yogurt Parfait

Ingredients:

- Greek yogurt
- Fresh berries
- Nuts (e.g., almonds or walnuts)
- Honey or maple syrup

Preparation:

1. Layer Greek yogurt into a bowl.

2. Top with fresh berries and nuts.

3. Drizzle with honey or maple syrup for added sweetness.

Cooking Time: No cooking is necessary.

2. Oatmeal With Nut Butter

Ingredients:

- Rolled oats
- Water or milk
- Nut butter options include almond or peanut butter.
- Sliced bananas

- Chia seeds

- Cinnamon

Preparation:

1. Cook rolled oats with water or milk according to package instructions.

2. Stir in a spoonful of nut butter until creamy.

3. Top with sliced bananas, chia seeds, and a sprinkle of cinnamon.

Cooking Duration: 5-10 minutes.

5. Smoothie with Greens:

Ingredients:

- Spinach or Kale.

- Frozen fruits (e.g., strawberries, bananas) - Greek yogurt or protein powder

- Almond Milk

- Peanut butter or avocado

Preparation:

1. In a blender, mix spinach or kale, frozen fruit, Greek yogurt or protein powder, almond milk, and nut butter or avocado.

2. Blend until smooth and creamy, adding additional almond milk as required to get the desired consistency.

3. Transfer the smoothie to glasses and serve immediately.

Cooking Time: No cooking is necessary.

6. Avocado Toast With Poached Eggs

Ingredients:

- Whole grain toast, avocado, poached egg, and sliced tomato.
- Sea salt, black pepper.

Preparation:

1. Toast the whole grain bread until it's brown and crispy.

2. Spread avocado over the toasted bread and sprinkle with sea salt and black pepper.

3. Finish with a poached egg and sliced tomato.

4. Serve immediately, sprinkled with more sea salt and black pepper as preferred.

Cooking Time: 10–15 minutes for toasting bread and poaching eggs.

7. Quinoa Breakfast Bowl

Ingredients:

- Quinoa - Water/milk
- Sliced fruit.
- Nuts, seeds, honey, or maple syrup.

Preparation:

1. Cook the quinoa with water or milk according to the package directions.

2. Place cooked quinoa in a bowl, then top with sliced fruit, nuts, or seeds, and a drizzle of honey or maple syrup.

Cooking Time: 15-20 minutes for cooking quinoa.

Recipes for Smoothies, Oatmeal, and Other Morning Meals

1. Berry Blast Smoothie

Ingredients:

- 1 cup of mixed berries (including strawberries, blueberries, raspberries)

- One ripe banana.

- Half cup Greek yogurt

-1/2 cup spinach

- One tablespoon of honey or maple syrup (optional)

- Half a cup of almond milk or water

- Ice cubes (Optional)

Preparation:

2. Combine all items in a blender.

3. Blend until smooth and creamy.

4. Add extra liquid as needed to get the appropriate consistency.

5. Pour into glasses and serve immediately.

Cooking Time: None (ready within minutes)

2. Peanut Butter Banana Oatmeal

Ingredients:
- 1/2 cup rolled oats
- 1 cup almond milk or water

- one ripe banana, mashed

- Two tablespoons of peanut butter

- 1 tablespoon honey or maple syrup (optional)

- A pinch of salt

- Sliced banana and cinnamon for topping.

Preparation:

1. In a saucepan, mix the rolled oats and almond milk.

2. Cook, stirring periodically, until the oats are soft and creamy, which should take around 5-7 minutes.

3. Add in the mashed banana, peanut butter, honey, or maple syrup (if using), and salt.

4. Continue cooking for an additional 1-2 minutes, or until well cooked.

5. Remove from the heat and transfer the oatmeal to serving dishes.

6. Before serving, garnish with sliced bananas and a sprinkling of cinnamon.

Cooking Time: 5 to 7 minutes

3. Avocado Toast with Poached Egg

Ingredients:

- 2 slices of whole grain bread, toasted

- One ripe avocado.

- 2 eggs

- Add salt and pepper to taste.

- Optional toppings include sliced tomato, arugula, and crushed red pepper flakes.

Preparation:

1. Preparation Time: 5 min.

2. Spread mashed avocado on toasted bread pieces.

3. Heat a saucepan of water to a medium simmer.

4. Crack the eggs into separate small dishes.

5. Carefully slip one egg at a time into the heating water.

6. Cook for 3-4 minutes, until the whites are set but the yolks remain liquid.

7. Remove the eggs with a slotted spoon and set them on top of the avocado toast.

8. Season with salt and pepper, then add any preferred toppings.

9. Serve immediately.

Cooking Time: 10-15 minutes, including poaching eggs.

4. Green Goddess Smoothie

Ingredients:

- 1 cup spinach

- 1/2 ripe avocado

- 1/2 cup frozen pineapple cubes

- 1/2 cup chopped cucumber.

- 1 tablespoon of fresh lime juice

- One tablespoon of honey or maple   syrup (optional)

- Half cup coconut water or water.

- Ice cubes (Optional)

Preparation:

1. Preparation Time: 5 min.

2. Combine all items in a blender.

3. Blend until smooth and creamy.

4. Add extra liquid as needed to get the appropriate consistency.

5. Pour into glasses and serve immediately.

Cooking Time: None (ready within minutes)

5. Overnight Chia Seed Pudding

Ingredients

- 1/4 cup chia seeds.

- One cup of almond or coconut milk.

- 1 tablespoon of honey or maple syrup.

- 1/2 teaspoon of vanilla essence

- Fresh fruit to top (e.g., berries, sliced banana)

- Nuts or seeds for topping (such as almonds or pumpkin seeds).

Preparation:

1. Preparation Time: 5 min.

2. In a dish or container, combine the chia seeds, almond milk, honey or maple syrup, and vanilla extract.

3. Stir thoroughly to mix.

4. Cover and chill overnight, or for at least 4 hours.

5. Before serving, mix the pudding thoroughly.

6. Add fresh fruit, nuts, or seeds as desired.

Cooking Time: None (overnight soak).

6. Veggie and Cheese Breakfast Quesadilla

Ingredients:

- Two whole-grain tortillas
- Two scrambled eggs
- 1/4 cup black beans (drained and rinsed)
- 1/4 cup chopped bell peppers.
- 1/4 cup shredded cheese (such as cheddar or mozzarella).
- Salsa and avocado slices to serve.

Preparation

1. Preparation Time: 5 min.
2. In a skillet, scramble the eggs until well done.
3. Remove eggs from the pan and put aside.
4. Place a tortilla in the skillet.
5. Place the scrambled eggs, black beans, chopped bell peppers, and shredded cheese on top of the tortilla.
6. Add the second tortilla on top.
7. Cook until the bottom tortilla is golden brown and crispy, then turn it and cook the other side.

8. Remove from the skillet and cut into wedges.

9. Serve with salsa and avocado slices.

Cooking Time: 10-15 minutes.

7. Banana Nut Breakfast Muffins

Ingredients:

- 1 1/2 cups rolled oats

- 2 ripe bananas (mashed)

- 1/4 cup honey or maple syrup

- 1/4 cup almond or peanut butter

- 2 eggs

- Add 1 teaspoon vanilla essence

- 1/2 teaspoon baking powder

- 1/2 cup chopped nuts (such as walnuts and almonds)

Preparation:

1. Preparation Time: 10 min.

2. Preheat the oven to 350°F/175°C and fill a muffin tray with liners.

3. In a mixing dish, combine the rolled oats, mashed bananas, honey or maple syrup, almond or

peanut butter, eggs, vanilla extract, and baking powder.

4. Fold in the chopped nuts.

5. Ensure you divide the batter evenly into the muffin cups.

6. Bake for 20 to 25 minutes, or until a toothpick inserted into the center comes out clean.

7. Let muffins cool before serving.

Cooking Time: 20 to 25 minutes

These dishes offer a variety of healthful and tasty choices for getting your morning started correctly. Enjoy! These dishes are intended to be quick and simple to make, so you can have a nutritious breakfast without spending too much time in the kitchen. Cooking times may need to be adjusted depending on individual tastes and kitchen equipment. Enjoy your tasty and nutritious morning meals!

Tips for Incorporating Lyme-friendly Ingredients

Lyme-friendly items should be included in your diet to help manage symptoms and promote overall health and well-being. Here are some recommendations for including these foods in your meals:

1. Focus on Fresh and Whole Foods

Choose fresh, whole foods whenever feasible. Choose organic fruits and vegetables to limit your exposure to pesticides and other contaminants. Incorporate a variety of colored fruits and veggies into your meals to guarantee you're getting a diverse range of nutrients.

2. Choose Lean Proteins

Add lean proteins to your diet, such as fowl, fish, tofu, tempeh, and lentils. These protein sources are less likely to aggravate inflammation than red meats and processed meats. To lessen the risk of foodborne disease, ensure that proteins are fully cooked.

3. Include Healthy Fats

Include healthy fats in your meals to promote brain health and minimize inflammation. Choose omega-3 fatty acid-rich foods such as fatty fish (salmon, mackerel, sardines), flaxseeds, chia seeds, and walnuts. Avocado, olive oil, and coconut oil are all great sources of healthful fats.

4. Emphasize Anti-Inflammatory Foods

Include anti-inflammatory foods in your diet to help manage the inflammation associated with Lyme disease. Antioxidant-rich foods include berries, leafy greens, cruciferous vegetables (broccoli, cauliflower, Brussels sprouts), and herbs and spices (ginger, turmeric, garlic).

5. Limit Sugar and Processed Foods

Reduce your consumption of sugar and processed meals, which can aggravate inflammation and impair the immune system. Instead, use natural sweeteners like honey or maple syrup, and if feasible, substitute whole grains for processed grains.

6. Be Aware of Food Sensitivities

Pay attention to how your body reacts to specific foods and components. Some people with Lyme disease may be sensitive or allergic to certain foods, such as gluten, dairy, or nightshade vegetables. Consider maintaining a food journal to monitor your symptoms and uncover probable causes.

7. Hydrate With Water

Maintain hydration by drinking lots of water throughout the day. Proper hydration is vital for detoxification and good health. Limit your intake of sugary and caffeinated beverages, since these might dehydrate the body and increase symptoms.

8. Experiment with Lyme-Friendly Recipes

Discover Lyme-friendly recipes and meal ideas to diversify your diet and make mealtime more pleasurable. Look for recipes that use nutrient-dense foods and emphasize health and energy.

9. Consult a Healthcare Professional

If you're not sure which items to include in your diet or have certain dietary limitations, speak with a healthcare expert or certified dietitian who specializes in Lyme disease. They may give tailored counsel and help based on your specific requirements and preferences.

10. Listen to Your Body

Finally, listen to your body and respect its requirements. Pay attention to how different meals make you feel, and then make decisions that promote your health and well-being. Trust your intuition and make diet modifications as needed to improve your overall health.

Lyme-friendly items in your diet can help manage symptoms and assist your road to healing and recovery. You may develop a healthy and supporting diet that promotes vitality and well-being by concentrating on fresh, whole meals, emphasizing nutrient-dense components, and remaining attentive to your body's specific requirements.

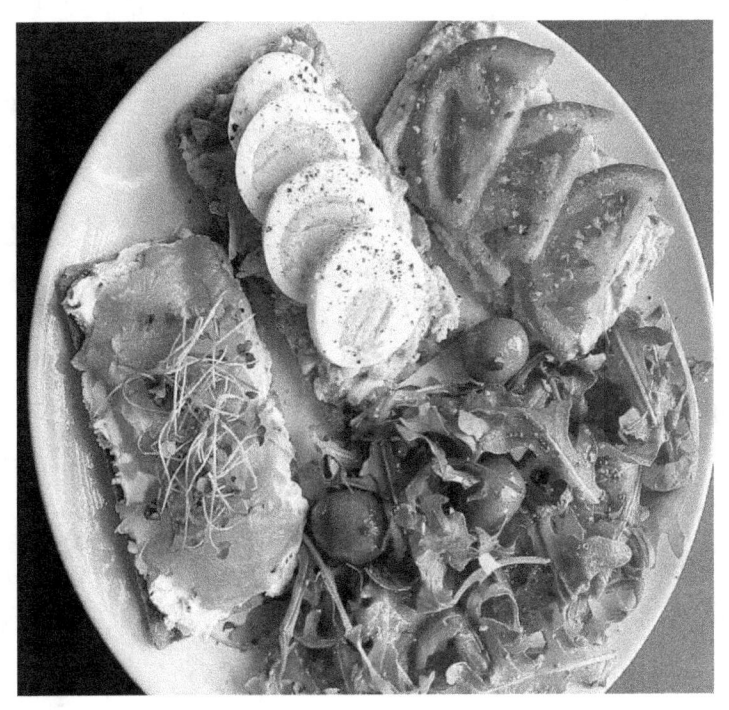

Chapter 4: Lunch Ideas

When dealing with Lyme disease, maintaining a balanced and nourishing diet is crucial to support the body's immune system and overall well-being. Lunchtime provides an opportunity to refuel with nutrient-dense foods that can help manage symptoms and promote healing.

In this section, we'll explore a variety of lunch ideas specifically tailored to individuals with Lyme disease. From vibrant salads to hearty soups and protein-packed wraps, these recipes prioritize ingredients that are gentle on the digestive system and rich in essential nutrients to support recovery and vitality.

Quick and Easy Lunch Recipes Suitable for Lyme Patients

1. Quinoa Salad with Mixed Vegetables

Ingredients:

- 1 cup rinsed quinoa
- 2 cups water or veggie broth
- 1 cup halved cherry tomatoes
- 1 diced cucumber
- 1 diced bell pepper
- 1/4 cup finely chopped red onion
- 1/4 cup fresh parsley, chopped
- Add 2 tablespoons of olive oil
2 teaspoons lemon juice.
- Add salt and pepper to taste

Preparation:

1. In a medium saucepan, heat the water or vegetable broth to a boil.

2. Add the quinoa, decrease the heat to low, cover, and cook for 15-20 minutes, or until cooked and liquid has been absorbed.

3. Remove from heat and allow it to cool slightly.

4. In a large mixing bowl, add cooked quinoa, cherry tomatoes, cucumber, bell pepper, red onion, and parsley.

5. In a small bowl, combine the olive oil, lemon juice, salt, and pepper.

6. Pour the dressing over the quinoa mixture and toss to incorporate.

7. Serve immediately, or chill until ready to eat.

8. Savor your healthful and tasty quinoa salad!

Cooking Time: 15-20 minutes.

2. Turkey and Avocado Wrap

Ingredients:

- Two big whole-grain tortillas.

Ingredients: 1/2 pound sliced turkey breast

- 1 mashed avocado

- One cup of baby spinach leaves

- 1/2 cup shredded carrots

-1/4 cup hummus

- Add salt and pepper to taste

Preparation:

1. Arrange the tortillas on a clean surface.

2. Spread the mashed avocado evenly on each tortilla.

3. Place turkey pieces, baby spinach, shredded carrots, and hummus on top of the avocado.

4. Add salt and pepper to taste.

5. Roll the tortillas firmly, tucking the edges in.

6. Cut each wrap in half diagonally.

7. Serve immediately or wrap in foil for a portable supper.

8. Savor your tasty, protein-packed turkey and avocado wraps!

Cooking Time: None.

3. Stir-fry with Chicken and Vegetables

Ingredients:

- 1 tablespoon olive oil

- 1 pound thinly sliced boneless, skinless chicken breast

- 2 cups mixed veggies (bell peppers, broccoli, snap peas, carrots)

- 2 minced garlic cloves

- 2 tablespoons soy sauce or tamari

- 1 tablespoon of honey or maple syrup

- One teaspoon of grated ginger.

- Serve with pre-cooked brown rice or quinoa

Preparation:

1. Heat the olive oil in a large pan or wok over medium-high heat.

2. Add the sliced chicken breast and simmer for 5-6 minutes, or until browned and well cooked.

3. Add the mixed veggies and garlic to the pan and cook for another 3-4 minutes, or until tender-crisp.

4. In a small bowl, combine the soy sauce, honey or maple syrup, and shredded ginger.

5. Pour the sauce over the chicken and veggies in the pan.

6. Stir well to evenly coat everything, then heat for a further 1-2 minutes.

7. Serve the chicken and vegetable stir-fry over cooked brown rice or quinoa.

8. Enjoy this delicious and nutritious lunch!

Cooking Time: 15-20 minutes.

4) Lentil and Vegetable Soup

Ingredients:

- 1 tablespoon olive oil
- 1 chopped onion.
- Dice two carrots and two celery stalks
- 2 garlic cloves, minced
- One cup of dry green or brown lentils, washed
- Add 4 cups vegetable broth
- 1 can (14 oz) chopped tomatoes
- 1 teaspoon dry thyme
- Add salt and pepper to taste
- Garnish with fresh parsley (optional)

Preparation:

1. Heat the olive oil in a big saucepan over medium heat.

2. Cook the chopped onion, carrots, and celery until softened, about 5-6 minutes.

3. Stir in the minced garlic and simmer for an additional 1-2 minutes.

4. Combine the washed lentils, vegetable broth, diced tomatoes, and dried thyme in the saucepan.

5. Bring the soup to a boil, then lower to a low heat and simmer for 20-25 minutes, or until the lentils are cooked.

6. Add salt and pepper to taste.

7. Serve the soup in dishes and sprinkle with fresh parsley, if preferred.

8. Savor this hearty and nutritious lentil and vegetable soup!

Cooking Time: 30 to 35 minutes

5) Tuna Salad Lettuce Wraps

Ingredients:

- Two cans of tuna (5 oz each), drained

- 1/4 cup mayonnaise or Greek yogurt

- One tablespoon of lemon juice

- 1/4 cup celery

1/4 cup chopped red onion

- Season with salt and pepper to taste

- Use butter lettuce leaves to wrap

Preparation:

1. In a mixing dish, combine the drained tuna,

Greek yogurt or mayonnaise, lemon juice, chopped celery, and red onion.

2. Season to taste with salt and pepper, then blend well.

3. Spoon the tuna salad mixture over the butter lettuce leaves.

4. Roll the lettuce leaves to make wraps.

5. Serve immediately, or chill until ready to eat.

6. Try these light and refreshing tuna salad lettuce wraps!

Cooking Time: None.

6. Hummus and Vegetable Plate

Ingredients:

- 1 cup hummus, either store-bought or homemade.
- Various raw veggies (carrot sticks, cucumber slices, bell pepper strips, and cherry tomatoes).
- Whole grain crackers or pita bread to serve.

Preparation:

1. Place the hummus in the center of a serving dish.

2. Serve the hummus with various fresh veggies and healthy grain crackers or pita bread.

3. Serve as a dip or spread for a fast and nutritious meal.

Cooking Time: None.

These lunch meals are quick to make and high in nutrients, making them ideal for people living with Lyme disease. Enjoy these tasty and nutritious meals!

Salad Ideas, Sandwich Alternatives, And Soup Recipes

1. Salad of Mediterranean Chickpeas

Ingredients:

- One 15-oz can of washed and drained chickpeas
- 1/4 cup finely chopped red onion
- 1/4 cup sliced Kalamata olives
- 1 cup chopped cherry tomatoes
- Two teaspoons finely chopped fresh parsley

- One tablespoon of lemon juice

- Two tablespoons extra virgin olive oil - One teaspoon dried oregano

- Season with salt and pepper

- Garnish with crumbled feta cheese (optional)

Preparation:

1. Combine the chickpeas, cucumber, red onion, cherry tomatoes, Kalamata olives, and fresh parsley in a big bowl.

2. Combine the olive oil, lemon juice, salt, pepper, and dried oregano in a small dish.

3. Drizzle the salad with the dressing and toss to fully incorporate.

4. If preferred, garnish with feta cheese crumbles.

5. When ready to eat, serve right away or store in the refrigerator.

6. Savor this tasty and revitalizing Mediterranean chickpea salad!

Preparation Time: None

2. Lettuce Wraps with Turkey and Avocado

Ingredients:

- A half-pound turkey breast cut into slices

- one sliced avocado

- 1/2 cup of carrots, shredded

- 1/2 cup of red cabbage, shredded

- Four big butter lettuce leaves

- 1/4 cup hummus

To taste, add salt and pepper.

Preparation:

Arrange the leaves of the butter lettuce on a sanitized surface.

2. Evenly distribute the sliced avocado, red cabbage, carrots, and turkey breast among the lettuce leaves.

3. Apply hummus to every leaf of lettuce.

4. To taste, add salt and pepper for seasoning.

5. To make lettuce wraps, roll up the leaves.

6. You can either eat right away or pack it in foil for a quick lunch.

7. Savor these nutrient-dense, light lettuce wraps with turkey and avocado!

3. Lentil and Butternut Squash Soup

Ingredients:

- One chopped onion
- One tablespoon of olive oil
- Two minced garlic cloves
- One chopped, peeled, and seeded butternut squash
- One cup of washed dry green or brown lentils
- 4 cups vegetable broth
- 1 teaspoon dried thyme
- To taste, salt and pepper
- Optional garnish of fresh parsley

Preparation:

1. Heat the olive oil in a big saucepan over medium heat.

2. Cook the minced garlic and chopped onion in the saucepan for about five minutes, or until the ingredients are tender.

3. Fill the saucepan with chopped butternut squash, vegetable broth, dry lentils, salt, and pepper.

4. After bringing the soup to a boil, lower the heat, and simmer it for 25 to 30 minutes, or until the lentils and butternut squash are soft.

5. Transfer sections of the soup to a blender and mix until smooth, then return to the pot, or puree the soup using an immersion blender until it's smooth.

6. Taste and adjust seasoning.

7. Spoon the soup into dishes and, if preferred, sprinkle with fresh parsley.

8. Savor this hearty and cozy soup made with butternut squash and lentils!

Preparation Time: 35 to 40 minutes

4. Salad Capers

Ingredients:

- Two big, sliced tomatoes
- One freshly sliced ball of mozzarella cheese
- Newly harvested basil leaves
- Two tsp balsamic glaze

To taste, add salt and pepper.

Preparation:

1. On a serving dish, arrange the mozzarella and tomato slices in succession.

2. Layer a few fresh basil leaves between the mozzarella and tomato slices.

3. Drizzle the salad with balsamic glaze.

4. To taste, add salt and pepper for seasoning.

5. Enjoy this traditional and reviving Caprese salad right away by serving it right now!

5. Hummus and Veggie Wrap

Ingredients:

- Two substantial whole-grain tortillas

- One cup of baby spinach leaves

- Half a cup of hummus

– 1/2 cup of carrots, shredded

- 1/4 cup of thinly sliced red onion

- 1/2 cup of thinly sliced cucumber

To taste, add salt and pepper

Preparation:

1. Evenly coat each tortilla with hummus.

2. Arrange sliced cucumber, sliced red onion, shredded carrots, and baby spinach leaves on top of the hummus.

3. To taste, add salt and pepper for seasoning.

4. Tuck the sides in as you carefully roll up the tortillas.

5. Cut each wrapper in half on the diagonal.

6. You can either eat right away or pack it in foil for a quick lunch.

7. Savor these savory and nourishing wraps with veggies and hummus.

Strategies For Packing A Lyme-friendly Lunch On The Go

Packing a Lyme-friendly lunch for when you're on the go is essential for maintaining a healthy diet and managing symptoms effectively. Here are some strategies to help you pack a nutritious and convenient lunch:

1. Plan Ahead

Take some time to plan your meals for the week, including lunches. Choose recipes and ingredients that are Lyme-friendly and easy to pack.

2. Choose Portable Foods

Opt for foods that are easy to transport and eat on the go, such as salads in a jar, wraps, sandwiches, and bento boxes with compartments for different foods.

3. Prep Ingredients in Advance

Preparing ingredients in advance can save time during busy mornings. Wash and chop vegetables, cook grains and proteins, and portion container snacks ahead of time.

4. Use Insulated Containers

Invest in insulated lunch bags to keep your food fresh and at a safe temperature while you're out and about. Consider using ice packs or frozen water bottles to cool perishable items.

5. Pack Nutrient-Dense Foods

Choose nutrient-dense foods that will provide sustained energy and support your overall health. Include a balance of lean proteins, healthy fats, fiber-rich carbohydrates, and plenty of fruits and vegetables.

6. Include Lyme-Friendly Snacks Pack snacks that are suitable for individuals with Lyme disease, such as nuts and seeds, fresh fruit, Greek yogurt, hummus with veggie sticks, and gluten-free crackers or rice cakes.

7. Avoid Common Triggers

Be mindful of common food triggers for Lyme patients, such as gluten, dairy, and processed sugars. Choose alternative ingredients and avoid processed foods whenever possible.

8. Stay Hydrated

Don't forget to pack plenty of water to stay hydrated throughout the day. You can also include herbal teas, coconut water, or infused water for added flavor and hydration.

9. Portion Control

Be mindful of portion sizes to avoid overeating and to ensure you're getting a balanced meal. Use smaller containers or portion out servings in advance to prevent overindulging.

10. Listen to Your Body

Pay attention to how your body responds to different foods and ingredients. Everyone's dietary needs are unique, so adjust your meals accordingly based on your symptoms and preferences.

By following these strategies, you can pack a Lyme-friendly lunch that supports your health and well-being while you're on the go. With a little planning and preparation, you can enjoy delicious and nutritious meals wherever your day takes you.

Chapter 5: Dinner Dishes

Preparing supper meals that are both delicious and appropriate for people with Lyme disease is critical for living a healthy lifestyle. Whether you're cooking for yourself or your family, supper is a time to eat nutritious and delicious meals that promote your overall health.

In this part, we'll look at a selection of supper recipes that are specifically designed to fulfill the nutritional requirements of Lyme sufferers. From tasty soups and robust stews to healthful grain bowls and protein-packed meals, these recipes highlight ingredients that are easy on the digestive system and high in crucial nutrients.

Nutritious Dinner Recipes For Satisfying Meals

1. Lemon Herb Baked Salmon

Ingredients:

- Four salmon filets (approximately 6 ounces each)

- 2 tablespoons of olive oil

- 2 cloves garlic, minced

- 2 teaspoons fresh lemon juice

- 1 teaspoon lemon zest

- 1 teaspoon dried thyme

- Salt and pepper to taste

- Lemon slices for garnish

- Fresh parsley for garnish

Preparation:

1. Preheat the oven to 400°F (200°C). Arrange parchment paper over a baking sheet.

2. Place the salmon filets on the prepared baking sheet.

3. In a small bowl, mix together olive oil, minced garlic, lemon juice, lemon zest, dried thyme, salt, and pepper.

4. Pour the lemon herb mixture over the salmon filets, covering them evenly.

5. Put a lemon slice on top of each filet.

6. Bake in the preheated oven for 12-15 minutes, or until the salmon is cooked through and flakes readily with a fork.

7. Garnish with fresh parsley before serving.

8. Serve the lemon herb baked salmon with your choice of side dishes, such as roasted veggies or quinoa.

Cooking Time: 12-15 minutes

2. Quinoa and Black Bean Stuffed Bell Peppers

Ingredients:

- 4 big bell peppers, halved and seeds removed
- 1 cup quinoa, washed
- 2 cups vegetable broth
- 1 can (15 ounces) black beans, drained and rinsed
- 1 cup of corn kernels, whether if it is fresh, frozen, or canned
- 1 cup chopped tomatoes
- 1 teaspoon chili powder
- 1/2 teaspoon cumin
- Salt & pepper to taste
- Shredded cheese for topping (optional)
- Fresh cilantro for garnish

Preparation:

1. Preheat the oven to 375°F (190°C). Grease a baking dish and arrange the bell pepper halves in the dish.

Heat the vegetable broth in a saucepan until it boils. Add the quinoa, decrease heat to low, cover, and simmer for 15-20 minutes, or until the quinoa is cooked and fluffy.

3. In a large bowl, add cooked quinoa, black beans, corn kernels, chopped tomatoes, chili powder, cumin, salt, and pepper.

4. Spoon the quinoa and black bean mixture into each bell pepper half.

5. Cover the baking dish with aluminum foil and bake in the preheated oven for 25-30 minutes, or until the bell peppers are soft.

6. If preferred, put shredded cheese on top of the filled bell peppers during the last 5 minutes of baking.

7. Garnish with fresh cilantro before serving.

8. Serve the quinoa and black bean filled bell peppers with a side of salsa or avocado slices.

3. Grilled Chicken and Vegetable Skewers

Ingredients:

- Cut two boneless, skinless chicken breasts into cubes.
- 2 bell peppers, cut into bits
- 1 red onion, cut into bits
- 1 zucchini, cut
- 1 yellow squash, sliced
- 8-10 cherry tomatoes
- 2 tablespoons of olive oil
- 2 cloves garlic, minced
- 1 teaspoon of dried Italian herbs, like basil, oregano, and thyme
- Salt & pepper to taste
- Wooden or metal skewers

Preparation:

1. If using wooden skewers, soak them in water for at least 30 minutes to prevent scorching.

2. In a large bowl, add cubed chicken breast, bell peppers, red onion, zucchini, yellow squash, and cherry tomatoes.

3. In a small bowl, mix together olive oil, chopped garlic, dried Italian herbs, salt, and pepper.

4. Pour the marinade over the chicken and vegetable mixture, stirring to coat evenly. Let the mixture infuse in the refrigerator for a duration of at least 30 minutes.

5. Preheat the grill to medium- high heat. Thread the marinated chicken and veggies onto the skewers.

6. Grill the skewers for 10-12 minutes, rotating periodically, or until the chicken is cooked through and the veggies are soft and slightly browned.

7. Remove off the grill and let them rest for a few minutes.

8. Serve the grilled chicken and veggie skewers with rice, quinoa, or a side salad.

Cooking Time: 10-12 minutes

4. Veggie Stir-Fry with Tofu

Ingredients:

- 1 block (14 oz) extra-firm tofu, cut into small pieces
- 2 teaspoons soy sauce or tamari
- 1 tablespoon sesame oil
- 1 tablespoon cornstarch
- 2 tablespoons vegetable oil
- 2 cloves garlic, minced
- 1 tablespoon grated ginger
- 2 cups mixed vegetables (like broccoli, bell peppers, snap peas, carrots)
- Cooked rice or noodles

Preparation:

1. Mix tofu with soy sauce, sesame oil, and cornstarch.
2. Cook tofu in a pan with vegetable oil until golden.
3. Add garlic and ginger, then mixed vegetables, and cook until tender.
4. Serve over rice or noodles.

Cooking Time: 15-20 minutes

5. Lentil Shepherd's Pie

Ingredients:

- 1 cup green or brown lentils
- 2 cups vegetable broth
- 2 tablespoons olive oil
- 1 onion, chopped
- 2 carrots, chopped
- 2 celery stalks, chopped
- 2 cloves garlic, minced
- 1 teaspoon dried thyme
- 1 teaspoon dried rosemary
- 1 cup frozen peas
- 4 cups mashed potatoes
- Salt and pepper

Preparation:

1. Cook lentils in broth until soft.
2. Sauté onion, carrots, celery, and garlic until soft.
3. Add herbs, cooked lentils, and peas, then season.
4. Transfer to a baking dish, top with mashed potatoes, and bake.

Cooking Time: 55-60 minutes

6. Mushroom and Lentil Pot Pie

Ingredients:

- 1 cup green or brown lentils
- 2 cups vegetable broth
- 2 tablespoons olive oil
- 1 onion, chopped
- 2 carrots, chopped
- 2 celery stalks, chopped
- 2 cloves garlic, minced
- 8 ounces mushrooms, sliced
- 1 teaspoon dried thyme
- 1 teaspoon dried rosemary
- 1 cup frozen peas
- 4 cups mashed potatoes or puff pastry
- Salt and pepper

Preparation:

1. Cook lentils in broth until soft.
2. Sauté onion, carrots, celery, garlic, and mushrooms until soft.
3. Add herbs, cooked lentils, peas, and season.

4. Transfer to a baking dish, top with mashed potatoes or puff pastry, and bake.

Cooking Time: 55-60 minutes

7. Lentil and Vegetable Casserole

Ingredients:

- 1 cup green or brown lentils
- 2 cups vegetable broth
- 2 tablespoons olive oil
- 1 onion, chopped
- 2 carrots, chopped
- 2 celery stalks, chopped
- 2 cloves garlic, minced
- 1 cup diced tomatoes
- 1 teaspoon dried thyme
- 1 teaspoon dried rosemary
- 1 cup frozen peas
- 1 cup grated cheese (optional)
- Salt and pepper

Preparation

1. Cook lentils in broth until soft.
2. Sauté onion, carrots, celery, and garlic until soft.

3. Add tomatoes, herbs, cooked lentils, peas, and season.

4. Transfer to a baking dish, top with cheese if using, and bake.

Cooking Time: 55-60 minutes

These nutritious supper ideas are not only tasty but also simple to make, making them excellent for hectic weeknights.

Main Course Options With A Focus On Lean Proteins And Vegetables

Here are some main course options suitable for individuals with Lyme disease, concentrating on lean proteins and vegetables:

1. Grilled Lemon Herb Chicken:

Ingredients:
- 4 boneless, skinless chicken breasts

- 2 teaspoons olive oil

- 2 cloves garlic, minced

- 1 teaspoonful raw lemon juice

- 1 teaspoon lemon zest

- 1 teaspoon dried thyme

- 1 teaspoon dried rosemary

- Salt and pepper to taste

Preparation:

1. In a basin, combine olive oil, minced garlic, lemon juice, lemon zest, thyme, rosemary, salt, and pepper.

2. Add chicken breasts to the marinade and marinate them well. Let them infuse in the refrigerator for a duration of at least 30 minutes.

3. Preheat the barbecue to medium-high heat. Grill the chicken breasts for 6-8 minutes per side, or until heated through.

4. Serve with a side of steamed vegetables or a mixed green salad.

2. Baked Salmon with Roasted Vegetables

Ingredients:

- 4 salmon filets

- 2 teaspoons olive oil

- 2 bulbs garlic, minced

- 1 teaspoonful raw lemon juice

- 1 teaspoon dried dill - Salt and pepper to taste

- Assorted vegetables (such as bell peppers, zucchini, cherry tomatoes)

Preparations:

1. Preheat the oven to 400°F (200°C). Put parchment paper on a baking sheet.

2. In a small basin, whisk together olive oil, minced garlic, lemon juice, dried dill, salt, and pepper.

3. Place salmon filets on the prepared baking tray. Use a brush to apply the olive oil mixture onto them.

4. Arrange the assorted vegetables around the salmon on the baking sheet. Pour any leftover olive oil mixture over them.

5. Bake for 12-15 minutes, or until the salmon is heated through and the vegetables are tender.

6. Serve the broiled salmon with caramelized vegetables alongside quinoa or brown rice.

3. Turkey and Vegetable Stir-Fry

Ingredients:
- 1 lb turkey breast, thinly sliced
- 2 tablespoons soy sauce
- 1 tablespoon sesame oil
- 2 cloves garlic, minced
- 1 teaspoonful minced ginger
- Assorted vegetables (such as broccoli, bell peppers, snap peas, carrots)
- Cooked rice or vermicelli for serving

Preparation:

1. In a basin, combine turkey slices with soy sauce, sesame oil, minced garlic, and grated ginger. Let them marinate for 15-20 minutes.

2. Warm a large skillet or griddle over medium-high heat. Add marinated turkey slices and stir-fry until cooked through, about 5-7 minutes.

3. Add assorted vegetables to the skillet and stir-fry until tender-crisp, about 3-4 minutes.

4. Serve the turkey and vegetable stir-fry over prepared rice or vermicelli.

4. Grilled Garlic Herb Shrimp

Ingredients:

- 1 lb large shrimp
- 2 tbsp olive oil
- 2 cloves garlic (minced)
- 1 tbsp lemon juice
- 1 tsp dried parsley
- Salt and pepper

Preparation:

1. Mix olive oil, garlic, lemon juice, parsley, salt, and pepper.

2. Toss shrimp in the mixture and let them sit for 15-20 minutes.

3. Cook the shrimp on the grill for 2 to 3 minutes on each side until they are fully cooked.

4. Serve with veggies or salad.

5. Baked Cod with Lemon Dill Sauce

Ingredients:

- 4 cod filets
- 2 tbsp olive oil
- 2 cloves garlic (minced)

- 1 tbsp lemon juice

- 1 tsp dried dill

- Salt and pepper

Preparation:

1. Preheat the oven to 375°F.

2. Mix olive oil, garlic, lemon juice, dill, salt, and pepper.

3. Brush mixture over cod filets.

4. Bake for 15-20 minutes until the fish flakes easily.

5. Serve with veggies or rice.

6. Stuffed Bell Peppers with Quinoa and Black Beans

Ingredients:

- 4 bell peppers

- 1 cup cooked quinoa

- 1 cup cooked black beans

- 1 cup diced tomatoes

- 1/2 cup diced onions

- 1/2 cup diced mushrooms

- Salt and pepper

Preparation:

1. Preheat the oven to 375°F.

2. Mix quinoa, black beans, tomatoes, onions, mushrooms, salt, and pepper.

3. Stuff bell peppers with mixture.

4. Bake for 25-30 minutes until peppers are tender.

5. Serve as a main dish.

7. Grilled Vegetable and Halloumi Skewers

Ingredients:
- Halloumi cheese
- Assorted vegetables
- 2 tbsp olive oil
- 2 cloves garlic (minced)
- 1 tbsp lemon juice
- Salt and pepper

Preparation:

1. Preheat the grill.

2. Thread cheese and veggies onto skewers.

3. Mix olive oil, garlic, lemon juice, salt, and pepper.

4. Brush skewers with mixture.

5. Cook on the grill for 3 to 4 minutes on each side.

6. Serve with couscous or salad.

These main course options provide lean proteins from chicken, salmon, and turkey, combined with a variety of colorful vegetables to create balanced and nutritious meals for individuals managing Lyme disease.

One-pot Meals And Slow Cooker Recipes For Convenience

For extra convenience, try these simple one-pot dinners and slow cooker recipes:

1. One-Pot Chicken with Rice

Ingredients:

- One pound of skinless, boneless chicken thighs

- One cup of rice

- Two cups chicken broth

- Diced onion

- Minced garlic cloves

- One sliced bell pepper

- One cup of frozen peas

- To taste, add salt, pepper, and your preferred herbs.

Preparation:

1. Brown chicken thighs on all sides in a big saucepan.

2. Cook the chopped garlic and onion until they become tender.

3. Add the spices, bell pepper, rice, and chicken broth.

4. Once the rice is done and the chicken is tender, decrease the heat, cover, and simmer for 20 to 25 minutes.

5. Before serving, stir in the frozen peas, cover, and allow to sit for a few minutes.

2.Beef Stew Made Slowly

Ingredients:

- 1.5 pounds of cubed beef stew meat

- 4 diced potatoes

- 2 sliced carrots

- 1 chopped onion

- Two minced garlic cloves

- 1 can of chopped tomatoes

- 2 cups beef broth

- A teaspoon of thyme, dried

- To taste, add salt and pepper

Preparation:

1. Fill a slow cooker with potatoes, carrots, onion, garlic, and beef stew meat.

2. Cover the items with diced tomatoes and beef broth.

3. Include the salt, pepper, and dry thyme.

4. After the veggies are well cooked and the meat is soft, cover and simmer on low for 6–8 hours or on high for 3–4 hours.

5. If preferred, top hot dish with fresh herbs.

3. One-Pot Vegetable Chili

Ingredients:

- One can of black beans that have been washed and drained.

- One can of washed and drained kidney beans

- Diced tomatoes, one can

- One chopped onion

- Two minced garlic cloves

- One sliced bell pepper

- One cup of corn, frozen

- Half a cup of chili powder, measured

- One teaspoon of cumin

- To taste, add salt and pepper

Preparation:

1. Saute the bell pepper, onion, and garlic in a big saucepan until they are tender.

2. Include the kidney and black beans, chopped tomatoes, frozen corn, cumin, chili powder, salt, and pepper.

3. Give it a good stir, put a lid on it, and simmer for 20 to 30 minutes to let the flavors blend.

4. Top with your preferred chili toppings, such as avocado, sour cream, or shredded cheese, and serve hot.

4. Slow Cooker Chicken Tacos
Ingredients:
- One pound of chicken breasts (no skin or bones)
- one package of taco seasoning.

- One cup salsa.

- One chopped onion.

- Two minced garlic cloves.

- One sliced bell pepper.

- One cup frozen corn.

- One can of black beans, cleaned and drained.

- Tortillas

- Optional toppings include avocado, sour cream, shredded cheese, sliced tomatoes, and lettuce.

Preparation:

1. Put the chicken breasts into the slow cooker.

2. Sprinkle taco spice over the chicken.

3. Combine the salsa, onion, garlic, bell pepper, corn, and black beans.

4. Set to low for 6-8 hours or high for 3-4 hours.

5. Using forks, shred the chicken and stir thoroughly.

6. Place the chicken taco filling in tortillas and garnish with any preferred toppings.

5. One-Pot Pasta Primavera

Ingredients:

- 8 ounces pasta (fusilli or penne

- 2 cups mixed vegetables (peas, carrots, broccoli, and bell peppers)

- 2 minced garlic cloves

- 1 cup coconut cream or heavy cream

- 2 cups vegetable broth,

- 1/2 cup grated Parmesan cheese,

- Salt and pepper to taste

-Fresh parsley or basil for decoration.

Preparation:

1. In a saucepan, combine the pasta, vegetables, garlic, cream, broth, and Parmesan cheese.

2. Season with salt and pepper.

3. Bring to a boil, then reduce to a simmer for 15-20 minutes, or until the pasta is cooked and the sauce has thickened.

4. Just before serving, garnish with parsley or basil leaves.

6. Slow Cooker Vegetable Curry
Ingredients:

- 1 chopped onion,

- 2 sliced carrots,

- 2 diced sweet potatoes,

- 1 diced bell pepper, and

- 1 can of rinsed and drained chickpeas.

- One can coconut milk.

- Use 1 cup veggie broth and

- 2 tsp curry powder

- One teaspoon of ground turmeric

- Season with salt and pepper to taste

- Use cooked rice

Preparation:

1. Place onions, carrots, sweet potatoes, bell pepper, and chickpeas in the slow cooker.

2. In a mixing bowl, combine the coconut milk, broth, curry powder, turmeric, salt, and pepper.

3. Pour mixture over vegetables.

4. Set to low for 6-8 hours or high for 3-4 hours.

5. Serve over rice.

7. One-Pot Garlic Shrimp Pasta
Ingredients:

- One pound large shrimp (peeled and deveined)
- Two tablespoons of olive oil
- 8 ounces of linguine
- four minced garlic cloves.
-one lemon(Extract the juice and zest the lemon)
- One-half cup heavy cream
- 2 cups vegetable broth
- Salt and pepper to taste
- Fresh parsley for garnish

Preparation:

1. Go ahead and heat the oil in a large skillet or frying pan.

2. Cook the garlic until it releases its aroma.

3. Combine the linguine, shrimp, lemon zest, juice, and broth.

4. Bring to a boil, then reduce heat and simmer for 10-12 minutes, or until the pasta is soft and the shrimp are cooked.

5. Stir in the cream, salt, and pepper.

6. Garnish with parsley and serve.

These recipes for one-pot dinners and slow cooker meals are ideal for hectic days since they require little preparation or cleanup time and still provide tasty, wholesome meals.

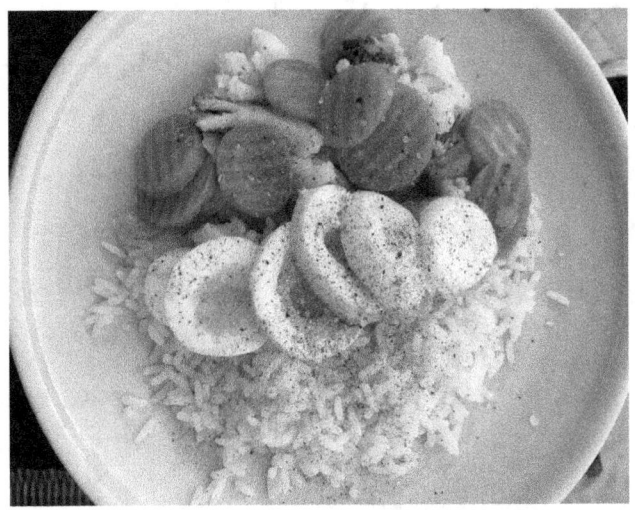

Chapter 6: Snacks and Treats

Managing Lyme illness while navigating snacks and indulgences may be pleasant and stressful at the same time. It's crucial to choose snacks that are satisfying, nutritional, and supportive of your health objectives. This section will look at many snack alternatives that are appropriate for those who have Lyme disease, with an emphasis on components that can help control symptoms and enhance general health. These snack options will keep you energized and satisfied throughout the day, without sacrificing your dietary requirements or health goals. They range from filling sweet sweets to bite-sized energy boosters.

Healthy Snack Ideas to Keep Energy Levels Stable

1. Nuts and Seeds Blended

Ingredients:

- 1/4 cup almonds

- 1/4 cup of walnuts

- Include 1/2 cup of pumpkin seeds

- Two tsp. sunflower seeds

Preparation:

Just combine the seeds and nuts in a dish.

2. Berries and Greek Yogurt

Ingredients:

- Half a cup of Greek yogurt

- 1/4 cup of mixed berries, including raspberries, blueberries, and strawberries

Preparation:

- Transfer the Greek yogurt onto a bowl, then sprinkle the mixed berries over it.

3. Vegetable Sticks with Hummus

Ingredients:

- Carrot sticks, celery sticks, and bell pepper slices;

- 1/2 cup hummus;

Preparation:

- Arrange the vegetable sticks on a platter for

dipping and place the hummus in a dish.

4. Nut Butter-topped Apple Slices

Ingredients:

- One sliced apple

- Two tablespoons of nut butter (peanut or almond).

Preparation:

- Drizzle the apple slices with the nut butter.

5. Roughly Cooked Eggs

Ingredients:

- Two eggs

Preparation:

- Put the eggs in a pan with water on top.

- After bringing the water to a boil, lower the heat, and simmer it for ten to twelve minutes.

- The eggs should be taken out of the water and allowed to cool before being peeled.

Preparation Time: 10–12 minutes

6. Energy Balls with Oatmeal

Ingredients:

One cup of rolled oats

- 1/4 cup honey

- 1/2 cup nut butter (almond or peanut butter)

- 1 teaspoon cinnamon

Preparation

-   In a bowl make sure you mix well all the combined ingredients

- Form the mixture into little balls that may be eaten.

- For added taste, feel free to roll the balls in cocoa powder or shredded coconut.

7. Mix for Trail Mix

Ingredients:

- 1/4 cup almonds

- 1/4 cup cashews

- Two tablespoons of sunflower seeds

- Two tablespoons of pumpkin seeds

- Two tsp of cranberries, dried

- Two tsp dark chocolate chunks

Preparation:

- In a bowl make sure you mix well all the combined ingredients

These quick and simple healthy snack alternatives are ideal for maintaining consistent energy levels throughout the day. Savor them as a component of a well-balanced diet to promote general health and wellness.

Lyme-friendly Desserts For Satisfying cravings

Try one of these Lyme-friendly dessert suggestions to satisfy your sweet tooth:

1. Cookies with Almond Butter

Ingredients:

- 1/4 cup honey or maple syrup
- 1 cup almond butter
- One egg
- one teaspoon of vanilla essence
- a pinch of salt

Preparation:

1. Preheat the oven to 350°F (175°C) and place parchment paper on a baking pan.

2. Thoroughly combine almond butter, egg, vanilla extract, honey or maple syrup, and salt in a bowl.

3. Scoop out bits of dough the size of a tablespoon and shape them into balls. Using a fork, flatten them after placing them on the baking pan.

4. Bake for ten to twelve minutes, or until the sides are browned.

5. Let cool completely before serving.

2. Avocado Mousse with Dark Chocolate

Ingredients:

- 1/4 cup chocolate powder

- 2 ripe avocados

- One teaspoon vanilla essence

- One-fourth cup honey or maple syrup - A pinch of salt

Preparation:

1. Scoop out the avocados' flesh and transfer them

to a food processor or blender.

2. Include salt, vanilla essence, honey (or maple syrup), and chocolate powder.

3. Blend, scraping down the sides as necessary, until creamy and smooth.

4. Before serving, transfer the mousse to serving plates and let it cool in the fridge for at least half an hour.

3. Popsicles with Coconut Berries

Ingredients:

- Mixture of berries (strawberries, blueberries, raspberries) and
- Two tablespoons of honey or maple syrup
- One tsp of vanilla extract

Preparation:

1. Put the mixed berries, honey (or maple syrup), coconut milk, and vanilla extract in a blender. Process till smooth.

2. Fill popsicle molds with mixture, insert sticks, and freeze until solid, at least 4 hours.

3. Submerge the molds in warm water for a brief period of time to release the popsicles.

4. Cookies with Banana Oatmeal

Ingredients:

- Two mashed, ripe bananas

One cup of rolled oats

- One-fourth cup almond butter
- 1/4 cup chopped nuts or chocolate chips, if desired

Preparation:

1. Preheat the oven to 350°F (175°C) and place parchment paper on a baking pan.

2. Put the mashed bananas, almond butter, rolled oats, chocolate chips, and almonds (if using) in a bowl.

3. Transfer dough sections, sized like a tablespoon, to the baking sheet.

4. Using a fork, flatten the dough, and bake for 12 to 15 minutes, or until golden brown.

5. Let cool completely before consuming.

5. Fresh Fruit and Chia Seed Pudding

Ingredients:

- One-fourth cup chia seeds

- One cup of coconut or almond milk

- One tablespoon of maple syrup or honey

- Half a teaspoon of essence from vanilla

- A variety of fresh fruit to garnish

Preparation:

1. Combine chia seeds, honey, maple syrup, almond milk, or coconut milk, and vanilla essence in a dish or container.

2. Put the pudding in the refrigerator, covered, and let it thicken for at least two hours or overnight.

3. Top with your preferred fresh fruit and serve.

6. Apple Cinnamon Energy Bites

Ingredients:

- 1/2 cup unsweetened applesauce

- 1 cup rolled oats

- One-fourth cup almond butter

- Two teaspoons of maple syrup or honey

- One teaspoon of cinnamon

- 1/4 cup dried cranberries or raisins (optional)

- A pinch of salt

Preparation:

1. Combine the rolled oats, applesauce, almond butter, honey, cinnamon, maple syrup, salt, and, if desired, dried cranberries or raisins in a bowl.

2. Using a tablespoon-sized rolling pin, roll the mixture into balls and arrange on a baking sheet covered with parchment paper.

3. Before serving, let the food cool for at least half an hour in the refrigerator.

7. Yogurt Bark, Frozen

Ingredients:

- Two cups of Greek yogurt

- One tablespoon of maple syrup or honey

- 1/2 cup of mixed berries, including raspberries, blueberries, and strawberries

- Two teaspoons of finely chopped nuts or seeds (almonds, walnuts, pumpkin seeds)

- Two tablespoons of optionally shredded coconut

Preparation:

1. Spread parchment paper on a baking sheet.

2. Thoroughly blend Greek yogurt with honey or maple syrup in a bowl.

3. Evenly distribute the yogurt mixture over the baking sheet that has been ready.

4. Evenly scatter chopped nuts or seeds, shredded coconut, and mixed berries on top of the yogurt.

5. Freeze the baking sheet for a minimum of two hours, or until the yogurt is fully solid.

6. Cut the frozen yogurt bark into chunks and savor it as a cool snack.

Tips for Managing Sugar Cravings While Adhering to Dietary Restrictions

Managing sugar cravings can be challenging, especially when following dietary restrictions such as those necessary for managing Lyme disease. However, with mindful strategies and healthy alternatives, it's possible to satisfy cravings without compromising health goals. Here are some tips for managing sugar cravings while adhering to dietary restrictions:

1. Understand the Cravings

Before addressing sugar cravings, it's essential to understand why they occur. Cravings can be triggered by various factors, including hormonal fluctuations, stress, inadequate sleep, and restrictive diets. By identifying the root cause of cravings, it becomes easier to develop effective strategies for managing them.

2. Stay Hydrated

Dehydration can sometimes mimic feelings of hunger or cravings for sugar. Ensure adequate hydration throughout the day by drinking plenty of water. Herbal teas and infused water can also be refreshing alternatives that help curb cravings.

3. Eat Balanced Meals

Consuming balanced meals that include a combination of protein, healthy fats, fiber, and complex carbohydrates can help stabilize blood sugar levels and prevent sudden spikes and crashes that trigger cravings. Focus on nutrient-dense whole foods such as lean proteins, vegetables, fruits, whole grains, and legumes.

4. Include Protein and Healthy Fats

Protein and healthy fats are satiating nutrients that help keep you feeling full and satisfied for longer periods, reducing the likelihood of sugar cravings. Incorporate sources of protein such as poultry, fish, tofu, eggs, and legumes, as well as healthy fats from avocados, nuts, seeds, and olive oil into your meals and snacks.

5. Choose Low-Glycemic Options

Opt for low-glycemic foods that have a slower impact on blood sugar levels, helping to prevent sugar cravings and maintain steady energy levels. Examples of low-glycemic foods include non-starchy vegetables, berries, nuts, seeds, whole grains like quinoa and barley, and legumes.

6. Sweeten Naturally

When cravings strike, satisfy your sweet tooth with natural sweeteners that offer some nutritional benefits without causing rapid spikes in blood sugar. Stevia, monk fruit, raw honey, and maple syrup are all viable alternatives to refined sugar. Be mindful of portion sizes and use these sweeteners sparingly.

7. Incorporate Fiber-Rich Foods

Fiber-rich foods help slow down the absorption of sugar in the bloodstream, promoting sustained energy levels and reducing cravings. Ensure to include plenty of fiber-rich fruits, vegetables, whole grains, and legumes in your diet. Snacking on raw veggies with hummus or fruit with nut butter can be satisfying options.

8. Plan Ahead

Having nutritious snacks readily available can help prevent impulsive choices when cravings strike. Prepare healthy snacks in advance and keep them easily accessible. Portable options like trail mix, homemade energy balls, sliced vegetables with dip, or Greek yogurt with fruit can be convenient choices.

9. Practice Mindful Eating

Pay attention to your body's hunger and fullness cues, and practice mindful eating to prevent mindless snacking and overindulgence. Eat slowly, savor each bite, and focus on the sensory experience of eating. Mindful eating can help you better regulate food intake and reduce the likelihood of succumbing to sugar cravings.

10. Address Underlying Stress

Stress can significantly impact cravings and lead to emotional eating behaviors. Find healthy ways to manage stress, such as practicing relaxation techniques, engaging in physical activity, spending time in nature, or seeking support from friends, family, or a mental health professional.

By implementing these strategies, you can effectively manage sugar cravings while adhering to dietary restrictions associated with Lyme disease.

Remember that it's essential to find a balance that works for you and prioritize overall health and well-being.

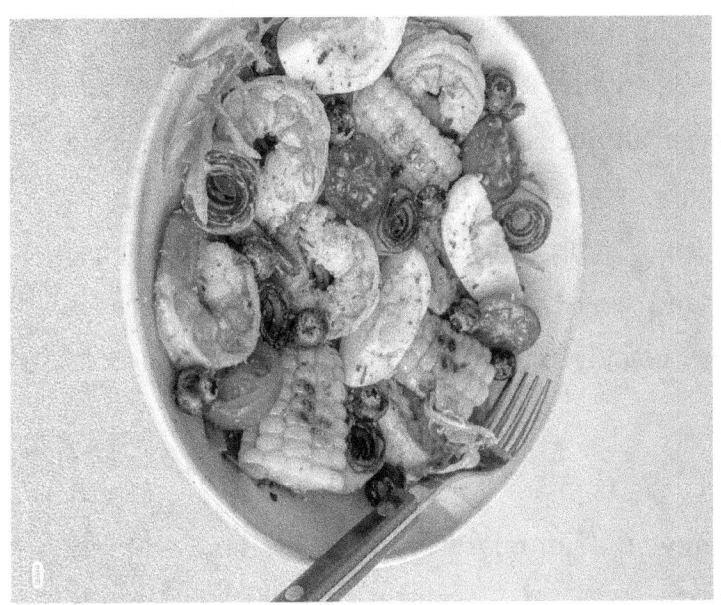

Chapter 7: Beverages To Support General Well-being

Lyme disease, a bacterial illness spread through the bite of infected ticks, can lead to a range of symptoms involving multiple body systems. While beverages alone cannot fix Lyme disease, picking the right drinks can play a supportive role in controlling symptoms and promoting general health and well-being. Here are several beverages that may be helpful for people with Lyme disease:

1. Water

Water is the basis of good health and hydration. It helps move nutrients, flush out toxins, control body temperature, and support different bodily processes. For individuals with Lyme disease, staying properly hydrated is important, especially since signs like fever, sweating, and increased urination can lead to fluid loss. Aim to drink at least 8-10 glasses of water per day, or more if you're physically busy or having signs like fever or diarrhea.

2. Herbal Teas

Herbal teas offer a soothing and hydrating choice with possible health benefits. Chamomile tea, known for its calming effects, may help reduce stress and promote relaxation, which can be helpful for people handling Lyme-related symptoms like anxiety and sleep disturbances. Ginger tea is another excellent choice, as ginger is well-known for its anti-inflammatory and stomach qualities. It can help reduce nausea, bloating, and gastrointestinal discomfort typically experienced by individuals with Lyme disease.

3. Bone Broth

Bone broth is a nutrient-dense beverage made by boiling bones and connective tissue in water for an extended time. It's rich in collagen, amino acids, vitamins, and minerals, including calcium, magnesium, and phosphorus. Drinking bone broth can support gut health, reduce inflammation, boost the immune system, and promote healing, making it especially helpful for people with Lyme disease. It's gentle on the digestive system and easy to digest, making it ideal for those having digestive problems or loss of appetite.

4. Green Juices

Fresh green drinks made from leafy greens like kale, spinach, and cucumber are packed with vitamins, minerals, antioxidants, and phytonutrients that can support general health and well-being. These nutrient-dense drinks provide hydration and help lower inflammation, detoxify the body, and boost immunity. Adding ingredients like ginger, lemon, and turmeric to green juices can improve their anti-inflammatory and immune-boosting qualities. However, be wary of fruit juices, as they can be high in sugar and may worsen symptoms like tiredness and brain fog.

5. Coconut Water

Coconut water is a natural and refreshing beverage that's rich in electrolytes like potassium, magnesium, sodium, and calcium. It's low in calories, fat-free, and naturally hydrating, making it an excellent choice for individuals with Lyme disease, especially those having signs like tiredness, muscle cramps, or dehydration. Coconut water can help restore electrolytes lost through sweating or sickness and support hydration and general well-being.

6. Probiotic Beverages

Probiotic-rich drinks like kefir, kombucha, and fermented coconut water contain helpful bacteria that can help promote gut health and support immune function. These probiotic drinks contain live cultures of bacteria that can help restore balance to the gut microbiome, which may be upset due to antibiotic treatment for Lyme disease. By supporting digestive health and immune function, probiotic beverages can help people with Lyme disease better control symptoms and improve general health and well-being.

7. Anti-Inflammatory Smoothies

Smoothies made with nutrient-rich ingredients like leafy greens, berries, avocado, and flaxseeds can provide a handy and delicious way to support health and well-being for people with Lyme disease. These drinks are packed with antioxidants, fiber, vitamins, and minerals that help lower inflammation, support immune function, and promote general health. Adding ingredients like turmeric, ginger, and cinnamon can further improve their anti-inflammatory qualities and provide additional health benefits.

Incorporating these drinks into your daily routine can help support your general health and well-being while handling Lyme disease symptoms. However, it's important to listen to your body and choose drinks that make you feel good and support your individual health needs. Additionally, speak with a healthcare provider or registered dietitian for personalized dietary advice tailored to your individual situation and symptoms. By focusing on hydration and nutrient-rich drinks, you can support your body's natural healing process and improve your health while living with Lyme disease.

Hydration Tips for Lyme Patients

Hydration is crucial for everyone, but it's especially important for people with Lyme disease. Proper water supports general health and well-being, helps clean out toxins, aids digestion, and supports immune function. Here are some hydration tips directly geared to Lyme patients:

1. Drink Plenty of Water

Water is the best way to stay fresh. Aim to drink at least 8-10 glasses of water per day, or more if you're physically busy, having symptoms like fever, sweating, or diarrhea, or if you live in a hot environment. Carrying a reusable water bottle with you throughout the day can help you stay hydrated more easily.

2. Monitor Your Urine Color

One way to gauge your hydration state is by tracking the color of your urine. Pale or light yellow urine usually indicates that you're well-hydrated, while dark yellow or amber-colored urine may suggest dehydration. Aim for pale yellow pee as a sign of proper hydration.

3. Add Electrolytes

Electrolytes are minerals like sodium, potassium, magnesium, and calcium that play important roles in hydration, muscle function, and nerve signals. When you sweat or lose fluids due to illness or drug side effects, you also lose electrolytes. Consider adding electrolyte-rich beverages like coconut water or sports drinks to your hydration routine, especially if you're sweating heavily or having signs like muscle cramps or tiredness.

4. Choose Hydrating Foods

In addition to drinking water, you can also improve

your hydration by consuming water-rich foods like fruits and veggies. Cucumbers, watermelon, oranges, strawberries, and cabbage are all examples of foods with high water content that can add to your general hydration levels. Soups, smoothies, and broths are also excellent choices for improving hydration while giving important nutrients.

5. Avoid Dehydrating Beverages

Some beverages can add to dehydration, so it's important to limit or avoid them, especially if you're prone to dehydration due to Lyme disease symptoms. Beverages like caffeinated drinks (coffee, tea, energy drinks), sugary sodas, and alcoholic beverages can have diuretic effects, increasing pee output and possibly leading to dehydration. If you choose to consume these drinks, do so in moderation and balance them with plenty of water.

6. Set Hydration Reminders

If you have trouble remembering to drink water throughout the day, try setting hydration notes on your phone or using a hydration tracking app. These reminders can help prompt you to take regular sips of water and ensure that you're keeping properly hydrated, especially during busy or stressful times when hydration may be overlooked.

7. Listen to Your Body

Pay attention to your body's signs and cues for thirst and water. Thirst is your body's way of telling that it needs more fluids, so don't ignore it. If you're feeling thirsty, tired, dizzy, or having symptoms like dry mouth or headaches, it may be a sign that you need to drink more water.

8. Hydrate Before, During, and After Physical Activity

If you're jogging or engaging in physical exercise, it's important to drink properly to replace fluids lost through sweat. Drink water before, during, and after exercise to keep hydration levels and support performance and healing. If you're practicing outdoors or in hot weather, be especially careful about staying hydrated and take frequent water breaks.

9. Consult with Your Healthcare Provider

If you have specific health concerns or medical conditions linked to Lyme disease, such as gastrointestinal problems or drug side effects, speak with your healthcare provider or a trained dietitian for personalized hydration suggestions. They can provide advice suited to your individual needs and help you create a hydration plan that supports your health and well-being.

By following these hydration tips and making hydration a focus in your daily routine, you can support your general health and well-being while handling Lyme disease symptoms. Remember that staying properly hydrated is important for improving your body's natural healing processes, supporting immune function, and boosting general health and vigor.

Recipes For Refreshing Drinks and Herbal Teas

Here are some recipes for herbal teas and cool drinks:

1. Lemon Ginger Detox Water

Ingredients:

- One sliced lemon and
- a one-inch piece of fresh ginger
- Four to six cups of water
- Ice cubes, if desired

Preparation:

1. Pour water into a pitcher.
2. Include the ginger and lemon slices in the water.
3. To let the flavors seep in, refrigerate for at least one or two hours.
4. If preferred, serve with ice cubes on top.

2. Mint Cucumber Cooler

Preparation:

- One cucumber, cut.
- Scoop of mint leaves that are fresh

- Four to six cups of water

- Ice cubes, if desired

Preparation:

1. Put cucumber slices and fresh mint leaves in a pitcher.

2. Pour water into the pitcher.

3. To give the flavors time to combine, refrigerate for a minimum of one hour.

4. For an even more refreshing beverage, serve over ice cubes.

3. Hibiscus Iced Tea

Ingredients:

- Two bags of hibiscus tea

- Four glasses of boiling water

- Optional honey or agave syrup

- Slices of lemon (optional)

Preparation:

1. Transfer the bags of hibiscus tea into a heat-resistant pitcher.

2. Cover the tea bags with boiling water and steep

for five to ten minutes.

3. Take out and throw away the tea bags.

4. If preferred, sweeten the tea with agave syrup or honey.

5. Chill in the refrigerator until ready to use.

6. Garnish with lemon slices and serve over ice.

4. Lavender and Chamomile Tea

Preparation:

- Two bags of chamomile tea

- One teaspoon of lavender buds, dried

- Four cups of boiling water

- Optional honey

Preparation:

1. Fill a teapot or heat proof pitcher with the dried lavender buds and chamomile tea bags.

2. Cover the tea bags and lavender buds with boiling water.

3. Steep for ten to fifteen minutes.

4. Take out the lavender buds and tea bags.

5. If desired, sweeten with honey.

6. Before pouring over ice, serve hot or chill in the fridge.

5. Tea with Ginger and Turmeric
Ingredients:

- A cut 1-inch piece of fresh ginger

- One teaspoon of ground turmeric

- Four cups of water

- Optional: honey or maple syrup

- Slices of lemon (optional)

Preparation:

1. Place the water, ground turmeric, and sliced ginger in a saucepan.

2. Heat the mixture over medium heat until it begins to simmer.

3. Simmer for ten to fifteen minutes.

4. Pour the tea into individual mugs.

5. If preferred, sweeten with honey or maple syrup.

6. Garnish with lemon slices if you want to.

6. Minty Green Tea Lemonade
Ingredients:

- 2 green tea bags

- 4 cups of boiling water

- 1/4 cup fresh mint leaves

- Quarter cup freshly squeezed lemon juice

- Two tablespoons honey or agave syrup (optional)

- Ice cubes

Preparation:

1. Allow the green tea bags to steep in hot water for 3-5 minutes.

2. Remove the tea bags and allow the tea cool to room temperature.

3. In a blender, mix the brewed green tea, fresh mint leaves, lemon juice, and honey or agave syrup.

4. Blend until the mint leaves are finely minced and the mixture is properly blended.

5. Strain the mixture through a fine mesh sieve to remove any solids.

6. Serve the minty green tea lemonade over ice cubes.

7. Raspberry Hibiscus Iced Tea

Ingredients:

- 2 hibiscus tea bags

- 1 cup fresh raspberries

- 4 cups of boiling water

- Honey or agave syrup (optional)

- Lemon slices (optional)

Preparation:

1. Place the hibiscus tea bags and fresh raspberries in a heat proof pitcher.

2. Pour boiling water over the tea bags and raspberries.

3. Let steep for 10-15 minutes.

4. Remove the tea bags and gently crush the raspberries with a spoon to unleash their flavor.

5. Sweeten the tea with honey or agave syrup if preferred.

6. Refrigerate until cool.

7. Serve over ice with lemon slices for garnish.

In addition to being delicious, these reviving beverages and herbal teas offer hydration and possible health advantages. Savor them all day long to keep yourself feeling renewed and invigorated.

How to Incorporate Lyme-friendly Beverages Into Daily Routines

Incorporating Lyme-friendly drinks into your daily routine can be a simple yet effective strategy to promote your general health and well-being while managing symptoms. Whether you're searching for hydration, nutrition, or a dose of antioxidants, there are lots of alternatives to pick from. Here's how to include these beverages into your everyday routines:

1. Start Your Day with Lemon Water
Squeeze fresh lemon juice into a glass of warm water each morning. This simple drink can help alkalize the body, assist digestion, and give a burst of vitamin C to strengthen your immune system.

2. Enjoy Herbal Teas Throughout the Day
Stock up on a range of herbal teas, such as chamomile, peppermint, ginger, and rooibos. These caffeine-free choices can help induce relaxation, calm digestion, and give antioxidant benefits.

3. Hydrate with Infused Water

Infuse your water with slices of cucumber, lemon, lime, or fresh herbs like mint or basil. This offers a refreshing flavor without any additional sweets or artificial additives, making it a perfect choice for remaining hydrated throughout the day.

4. Sip on Green Smoothies

Blend together leafy greens like spinach or kale with fruits such as berries, bananas, and mangoes for a nutrient-packed green smoothie. You may also toss in ingredients like chia seeds, flaxseeds, or nut butter for added protein and healthy fats.

5. Try Nutrient-Dense Juices

Invest in a decent juicer and experiment with creating your own nutrient-dense juices at home. Incorporate a variety of fruits and vegetables, such as carrots, beets, apples, and leafy greens, to produce tasty and healthful mixtures.

6. Opt for Homemade Broths & Soups

Make your own bone broth or vegetable broth to enjoy as a warming and hydrating beverage. You may sip on these nutrient-rich broths throughout the day or use them as a foundation for soups and stews.

7. Include Healing Tonics

Incorporate healing tonics into your regimen by combining ingredients like apple cider vinegar, honey, ginger, and turmeric with warm water. These tonics can help promote digestion, decrease inflammation, and enhance immunity.

8. Experiment with Adaptogenic Elixirs

Explore adaptogenic herbs like ashwagandha, rhodiola, and holy basil by putting them into elixirs or blended drinks. These herbs can help the body adapt to stress and improve overall balance and vigor.

9. Indulge in Decaffeinated Coffee Alternatives

If you appreciate the ritual of coffee but wish to

minimize caffeine intake, consider trying decaffeinated coffee alternatives like chicory root or dandelion root coffee. These choices deliver a comparable rich flavor without the stimulating effects of caffeine.

10. Stay Hydrated with Electrolyte Beverages

Electrolyte beverages can help replace important minerals and promote hydration, especially during periods of high perspiration or physical activity. Look for products that are minimal in sugar and free from artificial ingredients.

Incorporating Lyme-friendly drinks into your regular routines doesn't have to be complex. By focusing water, nutrients, and ingredients that promote your overall health, you may make tasty and pleasant drinks that add to your well-being. Experiment with different tastes and combinations to find what works best for you, and enjoy the benefits of remaining hydrated and fed throughout the day.

Chapter 8: Meal Planning and Tips for Success

Meal planning is a crucial aspect of maintaining a healthy lifestyle, especially for individuals managing Lyme disease. By taking the time to plan meals ahead, you can ensure that you're consuming nourishing foods that support your overall health and well-being.

Effective meal planning involves creating a menu for the week, considering dietary restrictions and preferences, and making a grocery list accordingly. It also allows for batch cooking and preparing meals in advance, which can save time and energy during busy weekdays. With thoughtful meal planning, you can set yourself up for success and make healthier choices effortlessly.

Strategies For Meal Planning With Lyme Disease

Meal planning can be particularly advantageous for

persons managing Lyme disease, as it allows for careful consideration of nutritional needs and symptom management. Here are some ideas for good meal planning with Lyme disease:

1. Start with a Balanced Diet

A healthy diet is vital for promoting general health and treating symptoms linked with Lyme disease. Focus on ingesting a range of nutrient-dense meals, including lean proteins, healthy fats, whole grains, fruits, and vegetables. Aim for colorful meals to guarantee a varied range of vitamins, minerals, and antioxidants.

2. Consider Dietary Restrictions

Many persons with Lyme disease may have special dietary limitations or allergies. Common limits include gluten, dairy, sugar, and processed meals. Take these limits into mind when planning meals and select for alternate items or substitutes to satisfy individual needs.

3. Plan Weekly Menus

Set some time each week to plan your meals for the future days. Consider things such as your schedule, available ingredients, and any special dates or events. Planning ahead helps you to build a cohesive menu that corresponds with your nutritional objectives and makes grocery shopping more effective.

4. Batch Cooking

Batch cooking entails making big quantities of food at once and portioning it out for many meals throughout the week. This strategy can save time and energy, particularly on hectic days when cooking from scratch may not be viable. Choose dishes that lend themselves well to batch cooking, such as soups, stews, casseroles, and grain bowls.

5. Include Lyme-Friendly Staples

Stock your cupboard and refrigerator with Lyme-friendly basics that form the backbone of your meals. This may contain products like lean proteins (chicken, fish, tofu), whole grains (brown rice, quinoa, oats), healthy fats (avocado, nuts, seeds), and lots of fruits and vegetables. Having these items on hand makes it easy to whip up healthful meals without much effort.

6. Focus on Quick and Easy Recipes

Opt for meals that are easy, quick to make, and need little cooking time. Look for one-pot meals, sheet pan dinners, and stir-fries that can be done in under 30 minutes. Additionally, try using kitchen equipment like slow cookers, Instant Pots, and air fryers to expedite the cooking process and save time.

7. Experiment with Meal Prep

Meal prep entails prepping ingredients or whole meals in advance to have on hand throughout the week. Spend a few hours on the weekend preparing veggies, marinating meats, and making grab-and-go snacks. Portion up meals into separate containers for convenient access during hectic weekdays.

8. Listen to Your Body

Pay attention to how different diets affect your symptoms and general well-being. Keep a food journal to chronicle your meals and any accompanying symptoms or reactions. This can help identify trigger foods or dietary patterns that increase Lyme disease symptoms, allowing you to make educated decisions regarding your diet.

9. Stay Hydrated

Adequate hydration is vital for sustaining overall health and wellness, particularly for persons with Lyme disease. Make sure to drink lots of water throughout the day and try including hydrating beverages like herbal teas, flavored water, and electrolyte-rich drinks into your meal plan.

10. Be Flexible

Flexibility is crucial when it comes to meal planning with Lyme illness. Symptoms might change, energy levels may vary, and unexpected occurrences can emerge. Be prepared to adjust your meal plan as required and give yourself grace on days when cooking feels tough. Remember that sustaining your body is a priority, and it's good to keep things basic when required.

By applying these methods, persons with Lyme disease may build a meal planning routine that supports their health, controls symptoms, and improves overall well-being. Experiment with different ways to determine what works best for you, and don't hesitate to seek help from healthcare experts or registered dietitians for individualized counsel.

Tips For Dining Out While Managing dietary Restrictions

Individuals with dietary restrictions, especially those with Lyme disease, may find it difficult to dine out. However, with proper preparation and discussion, you may enjoy meals in restaurants while adhering to your dietary requirements. Here are some guidelines for dining out while managing your dietary limitations.

1. Research Restaurants In Advance

Before going out to dine, spend some time researching restaurants in your region that cater to your dietary needs. Many restaurants now provide online menus, allowing you to browse the available meals and select products that meet your preferences. Look for restaurants that use fresh, whole foods and provide flexible menu alternatives.

2. Communicate Your Dietary Needs

When dining out, don't be afraid to disclose your dietary limitations to the restaurant personnel. Whether you have allergies, intolerances, or unique preferences, telling your server can assist guarantee that your food is cooked safely and according to your specifications. Be explicit and detailed about the items you must avoid, as well as any necessary adjustments.

3. Ask Question

If you have any questions regarding the ingredients or cooking techniques used in a certain dish, please do not hesitate to ask your server for an explanation. Inquire about how foods are prepared, whether particular components may be eliminated or swapped, and whether cross-contamination is an issue. Asking questions allows you to make better informed decisions and avoid potential triggers.

4. Look for Special Menus

Some restaurants provide customized menus or accommodations for guests with dietary requirements. These menus may feature gluten-free, dairy-free, or vegetarian alternatives, making it easier to select appropriate items without requiring substantial adjustments. When booking your reservation or dealing with your waitress, ask if there are any special meals or accommodations available.

5. Customize Your Order

Don't be hesitant to change your order to better fit your nutritional demands. Most restaurants are willing to allow replacements or alterations, such as changing ingredients, tweaking flavor levels, or removing specific sauces or garnishes. When making requests, be polite and considerate, and express appreciation for any adjustments made.

6. Focus on Simple Preparations:
When in doubt, choose foods with basic, easy preparations. Grilled, baked, or steamed foods are frequently safer options than fried or highly sauced dishes since they include less hidden components or allergies. Choose menu items that showcase fresh, whole foods and avoid meals with complicated sauces or spices.

7. Be Aware of Cross-contamination
Cross-contamination is a worry while dining out, especially for people who have severe allergies or sensitivities. When ordering, inquire about the restaurant's processes for preventing cross-contamination between items. Inquire about separate cooking surfaces, utensils, and preparation spaces to minimize allergy or trigger food exposure.

8. Consider Bringing Your Own Condiments

If you want to use special condiments or seasonings, bring them with you while dining out. This is especially useful if you are allergic or intolerant to common substances found in restaurant condiments, such as gluten or dairy. Just make sure to ask the restaurant personnel before using your own condiments at the table.

9. Practice Portion Control

It's tempting to overeat when dining out, especially if the meals are rich and indulgent. To avoid pain or worsening symptoms, use portion control and pay attention to your body's hunger and fullness cues. Consider splitting meals with dinner mates or requesting a half portion if available. In addition, aim to load your plate with nutrient-dense foods like lean meats, veggies, and whole grains.

10. Plan Ahead of Social Gatherings

Individuals with dietary limitations may face specific problems while attending social events or special occasions. If you want to attend a restaurant outing or an event, contact the host or organizer ahead of time to discuss your dietary requirements. Offer to bring a food to share that meets your requirements, or recommend eateries that provide adequate alternatives for everyone in the group.

Individuals with dietary restrictions, including those with Lyme disease, may dine out with confidence and enjoy excellent meals while prioritizing their health and well-being if they follow these guidelines. Remember to stand up for yourself, articulate your demands clearly, and make educated decisions that support your dietary objectives.

How To Adapt Recipes to Suit Individual Dietary Needs

Adapting recipes to meet unique nutritional demands can be beneficial for persons dealing with diseases such as Lyme disease, allergies, intolerances, or special dietary preferences. With some imagination and understanding of alternative products, dishes may be modified to meet varied dietary restrictions while still providing tasty and fulfilling dinners. Here are some recommendations for adapting meals to meet particular nutritional needs:

1. Understanding Your Dietary Needs

Before attempting to alter a dish, make sure you understand your dietary preferences and constraints. Take some time to determine which foods or substances you must avoid owing to allergies, sensitivities, or health concerns. Consider speaking with a healthcare practitioner or qualified dietician for specialized advice and suggestions.

2. Select Appropriate Substitutions

Once you've determined the components you should avoid, conduct study and choose appropriate substitutions that meet your dietary requirements. For example, if you are allergic to dairy, you can use plant-based substitutes such as almond milk, soy milk, or coconut milk in recipes.

Similarly, if you're on a gluten-free diet, choose gluten-free flours, grains, and starches such as rice flour, almond flour, or tapioca starch.

3. Experiment with Alternative Flour

For people with gluten sensitivity or celiac disease, replacing wheat flour with gluten-free alternatives is a typical solution. Try using almond flour, coconut flour, quinoa flour, or chickpea flour in recipes for baked goods, pancakes, or breading. Keep in mind that various flours may have distinct qualities that necessitate changes to the recipe's liquid or leavening ingredients.

4. Reduce the Sugar Content

Many recipes, particularly sweets and baked products, call for large amounts of refined sugars, which may be inappropriate for those with specific health issues or dietary choices. To minimize the amount of sugar in recipes, try substituting natural sweeteners such as honey, maple syrup, or dates. You may also experiment with lowering the quantity of sugar used in the recipe or adding mashed bananas or unsweetened applesauce for extra sweetness.

5. Increasing Fiber and Nutrient Density

Incorporate fiber, vitamin, and mineral-rich components into your meals to increase their nutritional worth. To improve fiber content and supply critical nutrients, include more vegetables, fruits, nuts, seeds, or whole grains in recipes wherever feasible. Add chopped veggies to soups, stews, and casseroles, or mix beans, lentils, or quinoa into salads and main courses to boost protein and fiber.

6. Focus on Whole, Unprocessed Foods

When modifying recipes, use entire, unprocessed ingredients wherever feasible. To prepare healthful and nutritious meals, use fresh produce, lean meats, and less processed grains and starches. Avoid highly processed or packaged foods, which may include additives, preservatives, or artificial components that might aggravate symptoms or cause allergies.

7. Mindful Seasoning and Flavoring

Pay attention to the seasonings and flavorings in recipes, since certain spices, sauces, and condiments may include allergies or trigger foods. To improve the flavor of foods, use natural herbs, spices, and aromatics rather than manufactured or packaged seasonings. Experiment with fresh herbs, citrus zest, garlic, ginger, and other natural flavor enhancers to give your dishes more depth and complexity.

8. Consider Food Sensitivities

In addition to allergies and intolerances, some people may have food sensitivities or special dietary preferences that impact the recipes they use. Take note of how specific meals influence your body and consider removing or decreasing those items from your recipes. Keep a meal journal to track your symptoms and discover probable triggers, then alter your recipes to improve your general health and well-being.

9. Practice Flexibility And Creativity

Adapting dishes to meet particular dietary demands necessitates culinary flexibility and innovation. Do not be hesitant to try new ingredients, methods, and taste combinations to see what works best for you. Accept the chance to explore new foods and dishes, and see adaptation as a means of culinary exploration and self-discovery.

10. Seek Inspiration and Resources

Finally, seek inspiration and tools to help you on your road to altering recipes to meet your dietary requirements. Look for cookbooks, recipe blogs, and food websites that focus on allergy-friendly, gluten-free, dairy-free, or plant-based meals. Join online networks or forums to interact with people going through similar dietary issues and exchange tips, advice, and recipe ideas.

Finally, adjusting recipes to meet specific dietary requirements takes careful planning, ingredient selection, and experimenting. Understanding your dietary limitations, selecting appropriate substitutions, and embracing creativity in the kitchen allow you to prepare tasty and enjoyable meals that promote your health and well-being. Remember to listen to your body, focus on full, unprocessed meals, and enjoy the journey of culinary discovery and adaptation.

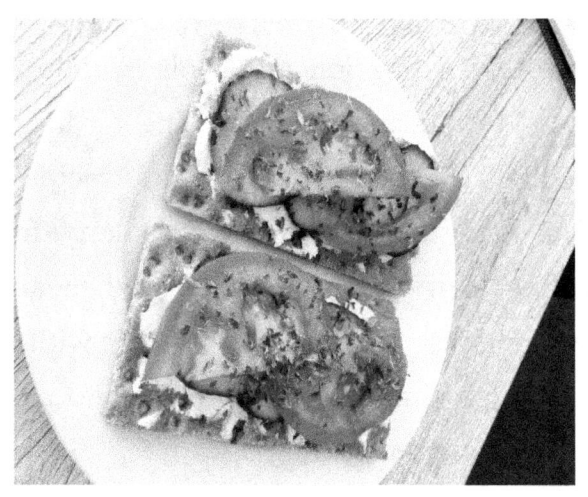

Conclusion

Managing Lyme disease with nutrition may be a difficult but rewarding process that needs commitment, patience, and a willingness to make lifestyle adjustments. While there is no one-size-fits-all method to controlling Lyme disease, eating a nutrient-dense diet can help you maintain your general health and well-being. You may improve your body's capacity to fight infection, reduce inflammation, and promote healing by concentrating on nourishing it with healthy diets, avoiding inflammatory triggers, and emphasizing nutrient-dense nutrients.

One of the most important concepts for controlling Lyme disease via diet is to eat full, unprocessed foods high in vitamins, minerals, antioxidants, and anti-inflammatory chemicals. Incorporating enough of fresh fruits, vegetables, leafy greens, lean proteins, healthy fats, and complex carbs into your diet can give your body with the important nutrients it requires to improve immunological function, reduce inflammation, and boost overall vitality.

When going on a nutritional path to treat Lyme disease, you must approach it with openness, curiosity, and self-compassion. Recognize that adopting dietary changes is not always simple, and it is okay to seek help from healthcare experts, registered dietitians, or support groups who may offer advice, encouragement, and practical recommendations along the way.

As you start your diet journey, here are some words of encouragement and guidance for beginners:

1. Start Slowly

Making substantial dietary adjustments at once might be daunting and unsustainable. Instead, gradually incorporate tiny, doable adjustments into your diet and lifestyle. Focus on implementing one new healthy habit at a time, such as adding more veggies to your meals, drinking more water, or replacing manufactured snacks with whole foods.

2. Listen To Your Body

Pay attention to how various meals make you feel and how your body reacts to diet changes. Keep a food journal to monitor your symptoms, energy levels, digestion, and general health. This can help you discover potential triggers, sensitivities, or trends that may be influencing your symptoms and direct your food choices appropriately.

3. Stay Educated

Learn about Lyme disease, its symptoms, and how nutrition and lifestyle can affect your health. Stay up to date on the newest research, nutritional methods, and evidence-based advice for controlling Lyme disease with food. Knowledge is power, and the more you understand about your condition and how to support it with diet, the more prepared you will be to make health-related decisions.

4. Find Your Support System

Surround yourself with a supporting network of friends, family, healthcare professionals, and fellow Lyme fighters who understand and sympathize with your experience. Share your experiences, struggles, and successes with others who can provide encouragement, guidance, and emotional support. Connecting with people facing similar circumstances may bring a sense of affirmation, friendship, and optimism.

5. Practice Self-Care

Dealing with Lyme disease can be physically, emotionally, and psychologically taxing at times. It is critical to emphasize self-care and participate in activities that feed your mind, body, and soul. Relaxation techniques, mindfulness, meditation, yoga, or light exercise can help you decrease stress, relax, and improve your general well-being. Remember to prioritize enough sleep, rest, and downtime to restore and renew your body.

Treating Lyme disease via nutrition is a process that involves patience, effort, and self-compassion. You may take charge of your health and well-being by concentrating on fueling your body with nutritious meals, listening to your body's signals, getting assistance from others, keeping educated, and prioritizing self-care.

Remember that every tiny step you take toward living a healthy lifestyle is a step in the right way, and every decision you make has the potential to improve your road to healing and recovery. You are not alone on this road, and with drive, perseverance, and support, you can overcome the obstacles of Lyme disease and live a life of energy and well-being.

www.ingramcontent.com/pod-product-compliance
Lightning Source LLC
Chambersburg PA
CBHW071044290526

45795CB00004B/1307